Praise for The Pain Antidote

"An authoritative, caring guide offering concrete suggestions—and hope—for anyone stuck in the tenacious grip of opioid pain medication addiction."
> —Sharon Wegscheider-Cruse, author and educator, and Joseph R. Cruse, MD, addiction medicine specialist

"Dr. Mel Pohl and Katherine Ketcham are intimately acquainted with chronic pain and know the road to freedom. This is the roadmap for anyone who wants their life back."
> —Debra Jay, author of *It Takes a Family* and *No More Letting Go*

Praise for Mel Pohl

"Dr. Pohl's quarter of a century as an addiction specialist, combined with his hands-on experience with patients teaching them drug-free solutions to their agony, and his five-year struggle to recover from his own terrible bout with pain give this book its unique perspective and authenticity . . . *A Day Without Pain* [offers] a realistic expectation of improved functioning, reduced pain, and more enjoyment of life."
> —HealthNewsDigest.com

Praise for Katherine Ketcham

"In the nearly 20 years since Ketcham coauthored *Under the Influence*, it has become a classic in identifying and treating alcohol addiction . . . This book offers a plethora of timely information; a blow to old stigmas, myths and stereotypes; and hope for a future in which many senseless tragedies can be avoided and lives saved."
> —Publishers Weekly on Beyond the Influence

ALSO BY MEL POHL, MD

A Day Without Pain

Pain Recovery
(with Frank J. Szabo Jr., LADC,
Daniel Shiode, PhD, and Robert Hunter, PhD)

Pain Recovery for Families
(with Frank J. Szabo Jr., LADC,
Daniel Shiode, PhD, and Robert Hunter, PhD)

ALSO BY KATHERINE KETCHAM

Beyond the Influence
(with William F. Asbury)

Teens Under the Influence
(with Nicolas A. Pace, MD)

Under the Influence
(with James R. Milam, PhD)

The Spirituality of Imperfection
(with Ernest Kurtz)

Experiencing Spirituality
(with Ernest Kurtz)

the

PAIN
Antidote

THE PROVEN PROGRAM TO HELP YOU STOP
SUFFERING FROM CHRONIC PAIN, AVOID ADDICTION
TO PAINKILLERS—AND RECLAIM YOUR LIFE

Mel Pohl, MD
and Katherine Ketcham

Da Capo
∞
LIFE
LONG

A Member of the Perseus Books Group

Designed by Trish Wilkinson
Set in 11-point Goudy Oldstyle STD by the Perseus Books Group

Library of Congress Cataloging-in-Publication Data

Pohl, Mel.
    The pain antidote : the proven program to help you stop suffering from chronic pain, avoid addiction to painkillers—and reclaim your life / by Mel Pohl, MD, and Katherine Ketcham.
        pages   cm
    Includes bibliographical references and index.
    ISBN 978-0-7382-1803-8 (paperback) — ISBN 978-0-7382-1804-5 (e-book)
1. Pain—Treatment—Popular works. 2. Chronic pain—Treatment—Popular works. 3. Pain medicine—Popular works. I. Ketcham, Katherine, 1949– II. Title.
RB127.P644 2015
616'.0472—dc23   2014049017

First Da Capo Press edition 2015

Published by Da Capo Press
A Member of the Perseus Books Group
www.dacapopress.com

Da Capo Press books are available at special discounts for bulk purchases in the U.S. by corporations, institutions, and other organizations. For more information, please contact the Special Markets Department at the Perseus Books Group, 2300 Chestnut Street, Suite 200, Philadelphia, PA 19103, or call (800) 810-4145, ext. 5000, or e-mail special. markets@perseusbooks.com.

10 9 8 7 6 5 4 3 2 1

Contents

How to Use This Book

WHO IS THIS BOOK FOR?

In short, *The Pain Antidote* is for anyone with chronic pain. When Kathy and I started to conceptualize this book a few years ago, our compelling intention was to reach out to a broad audience of people suffering with chronic pain.

Some of our readers will be using opioid drugs to relieve their pain. You may take them infrequently. "At most I take one or two Vicodin a day, exactly as my doctor prescribed for me, and in five years, I haven't increased the dosage—is this book for me?"

Perhaps you are taking high doses of multiple drugs. Your drug use may be causing problems for you, and you may know that you are dependent on the drugs for relieving your pain. "I need the drugs to relieve my pain, but am I addicted? How can this book help me?"

Or perhaps you do not take any opioid drugs at all. "Well, I took OxyContin when my doctor prescribed it, but I stopped years ago. Yet I still have pain. Why should I read this book?"

We wrote this book for all such readers—for anyone who lives with chronic pain. We also wrote this book for family members who seek to understand the nature of chronic pain and how to help their loved ones.

We wrote this book for physicians and other health-care professionals as well. Many doctors anticipate poor outcomes for their patients living with chronic pain and for their addicted patients. And yet for most physicians, these patients constitute a large percentage of their practices. Understanding how opioid drugs affect the brain and body helps dismantle many of the myths and misconceptions and clarifies the rationale for treatment methods and setting realistic goals. Reading the dozens of case histories in the pages that follow will help doctors and other health-care practitioners understand the devastating personal cost of chronic pain as well as the courage and determination required to learn how to live and thrive drug-free.

I have treated hundreds of people with chronic pain and watched them transform themselves from drugged, disabled, and depressed to alert, awake, and truly joyful for the first time in years. This is the closest thing to miracle work I've ever done in my thirty-eight years as a physician. I travel and lecture all around the country about this topic and after being away from the treatment center for three or four days, I can see the astonishing changes that take place in men and women, some in their teens and others in their eighties, who were once severely debilitated by physical and emotional pain. I'm greeted with smiles, laughter, hugs, and stories detailing their progress—and my heart swells.

WHAT WILL I LEARN?

You will learn that you can live a rich and full life with chronic pain. In these pages I share stories about the successes I have witnessed and offer details about the techniques and strategies that have proven most effective for people living with chronic pain. The program set forth in these pages is eminently practical and easily adapted to your individual lifestyle. Most important of all, these methods work. They can work miracles, if you do the work.

"Why do I have pain and why won't it go away? What's going on inside me?" you may be wondering. These questions are often expressed with a sense of hopelessness and despair. Being well informed about the nature of chronic pain will help you break through your confusion and fear. Thus, Part 1 focuses on the physiology of pain, the powerful role emotions play in chronic pain, and provides clear answers to questions about drug dependence and addiction.

In Part 2 you will find the most effective techniques and strategies, all of which you can learn and practice on your own, in your own home, to help you live and thrive with chronic pain. You will also find information and advice about professional therapies, such as acupuncture and physical therapy, with details about the basic philosophy and techniques to help you understand why these methods work for so many people in chronic pain.

The Jump Start plans detailed in Part 3 are packed full with practical and useful suggestions, and we devote an entire chapter to the connection between food and pain, again with practical, detailed information (and an appendix filled with dozens of healthy recipes). If you find yourself in a rut, this information will help you choose between the many options available to you to create week-by-week recovery and meal plans that you can proceed with at your own pace.

As you read this book, keep in mind that there is just one absolute requirement for this program to work for you: commitment. Throw yourself into the pages of this book, make a commitment to work the program set out for you, and have faith that the information and healing strategies you discover within these pages will make a difference in your life.

Because you can change your life. The antidote to chronic pain is within your reach. With awareness, courage, diligence, hope, faith, joy, compassion, and wonder, a new life full of meaning and purpose awaits you.

An important note about discontinuing medications: Throughout this book, we'll talk about life without painkillers. But *you must not simply stop your medications.* Over time, your body most likely has become accustomed to them and you may be physically dependent on them. Simply stopping these medications suddenly may be dangerous. You must consult a knowledgeable health-care provider or treatment center to supervise withdrawal from habit-forming medications, including opioids, sedatives, hypnotics, and alcohol.

Two more pieces of information for you:

We use the term *opioid* throughout the book because it is a more accurate representation of the terminology for narcotic painkillers than *opiate* (which is derived from the poppy plant that contains opium). Common opiates include morphine and codeine. An opioid is a substance (molecule) that is synthetic or partly synthetic, and not found in nature. The term *opioid* covers most of the drugs discussed in the book.

Second, most of the stories I will tell you are a composite of traits and experiences I've had with hundreds of patients over the past ten years. Kathy and I do tell actual patients' stories with their permission, of course, but have changed other names for the purposes of confidentiality.

Part 1

UNDERSTANDING

Your pain is the breaking of the
shell that encloses your understanding.

—KHALIL GIBRAN

In Part 1 you will learn about chronic pain, how and where it is generated in the brain, and why researchers believe it is a disease in and of itself. You will discover how fear, anxiety, anger, guilt, grief, and helplessness intensify chronic pain and why it is important to distinguish between pain and suffering. We will look at the drugs prescribed for chronic pain and the role these drugs can play in exacerbating—and even creating—chronic pain. And you will learn the distinction between addiction and dependence, which will answer one of the most oft-asked (and fear-filled) questions: "Am I addicted to—or just dependent on—the drugs I take to relieve my pain?"

Whether or not you are using opioid medications, the principles and techniques you will find in these chapters will help you live a better life with your pain.

ONE

ALL PAIN IS REAL

Everything You Wish You Never Needed to Know About Chronic Pain

Few experiences in life are more
universal than pain, which flows like lava
beneath the crust of daily life.

—PAUL BRAND AND PHILIP YANCEY

Loretta was complaining about her chronic pain. As I shifted in my chair, careful to keep my expression neutral, trying my best to hide my impatience and frustration, I found myself thinking that the words *whining* and *exaggerating* certainly applied.

"I have excruciating pain in my back." Loretta touched her lower back and grimaced, shifting her weight. "And in my neck." For perhaps the third time, she closed her eyes and bit her lip, as if to underscore the severity of her pain.

I found myself not liking her very much. I wanted her to go away. A voice inside me whispered, "So, what do you expect me to do about it?" After all, I was an addiction medicine specialist. My work was to help people get *off* drugs, but Loretta, like so many patients with chronic pain, wanted relief from the pain at any cost and that meant she wanted more drugs than I was comfortable giving her. She admitted she was addicted to drugs and reluctantly agreed to enter treatment to deal with her addiction because of the pressure from her concerned family members, but she also reiterated in a rising tone of voice that her pain was intolerable without drugs.

"You have to give me something to take this awful pain away! I'm begging you!" she said. I found myself tightening my jaw and noticed a throbbing ache in *my* low back.

"And my hands," Loretta said, gently rubbing her left thumb and index finger against the knuckles of her right hand, which were red and swollen. "My hands are killing me."

"Killing you?" I asked, careful to keep my tone even. Clearly she was in pain, but I knew it wouldn't kill her—what I needed to help her understand was the very real possibility that the drugs might. She was taking massive doses of painkillers: 10 mg of Vicodin, up to ten per day; 30 mg Percocet, six per day; and, depending on which doctor she saw that week, 80 mg of OxyContin or 60 mg of long-acting morphine three times per day. Her primary care doctor originally prescribed Vicodin and when that drug stopped working to relieve her pain even at higher doses, he referred her to a pain specialist who prescribed Percocet, then added OxyContin and, finally, long-acting morphine. She continued to visit her family doctor who dutifully prescribed 180 (10 mg) Vicodin per month, unaware of the magnitude of her opioid habit or the fact that she continued to get medications from her pain doctor and occasionally visited a local urgent care center or emergency room . . . where she was prescribed even more meds.

But at some point, even the morphine stopped working. In fact, she told me that she was in more pain than ever.

I pointed to the pain level chart prominently displayed in my office. "On a scale of 0 to 10, with 0 representing no pain and 10 being the worst pain imaginable," I asked Loretta, "how would you rate your pain?"

"Nine," she said, with no hesitation.

I consulted her file, flipping through the pages. "When you first went to your doctor for pain and started using Vicodin, what was your pain level?"

"Oh, maybe a 4 or 5," she sighed. "But it's gotten so much worse. I'm in agony. I can't live without my drugs. I'm miserable with them, but where would I be without them? I'd rather die than live with this pain."

I took a deep breath and mentally reviewed the facts of her case. As Loretta's tolerance increased, the drugs stopped working. Even steadily increasing doses of potent painkilling drugs didn't appear to touch her pain. In fact, her pain was worse than ever. From everything she was saying, it became clear that the drugs were adding to her misery on many levels, rather than subtracting from it. I had seen this before in many other patients. At these dosage levels, overdose was a real possibility and in the meantime, the drugs were gradually robbing her of all meaning in her life. She could no longer work as a grocery store cashier, her marriage was in serious trouble, her three adult children were so frustrated after years of listening to her complaints that they rarely called or visited, and her friends had "abandoned" her. She couldn't drive and was dependent on her husband for just about everything. She often spent the entire day in bed—even getting up to go to the bathroom was such a painful ordeal that her husband purchased a bedside commode. At forty-eight years old, she was, essentially, an invalid.

In the month before she voluntarily came to treatment, she had seriously contemplated suicide. "Sometimes I empty the bottle of pills into my hand and think about taking them all just to put an end to all our misery," she confessed. "But I'm too big a chicken."

Loretta's emotional state deeply concerned me, and I found myself wondering about the connection between the depth of her pain and the intensity of her emotions. As her pain increased, she admitted that she had become increasingly angry and depressed. Was it possible that her emotions were intensifying her pain, functioning as internal megaphones that amplified the "sound" of her physical pain?

MY EPIPHANY

And that's when the lightbulb came on. Loretta wasn't simply a complainer or a whiner. She wasn't exaggerating. She was in real pain. *Real* pain that wasn't being helped by the drugs she was taking; in fact, the drugs were making her pain worse. And she was suffering—mentally, emotionally, spiritually—as well. Her 9 on the pain scale was an accurate description of her overall experience of pain.

At that moment, almost a decade ago, something inside me shifted. Loretta's pain was real. Her suffering was real and was a substantial part of her overall experience of pain. It was not my job to judge or label her; in fact it was my job *not* to judge her. It was my responsibility to help her as best I could, and I wasn't going to be much help if I did what so many other doctors had done, and just passed her down the line— treating her addiction, assuring her that I had done all I could do, and referring her right back to her primary care doctor, a specialist, or a pain

clinic. Loretta would go full circle and end up right where she was before she came to treatment, except even more frustrated and depressed.

I knew from experience that most doctors treat chronic pain with
opioid drugs, increasing the dosages in a well-intentioned effort to reduce the pain. Or they refer their chronic pain patients to pain specialists who may prescribe even stronger drugs, adding anxiety meds
and sedatives to the painkiller mix. The patient might be scheduled
for a series of cortisone injections into the spine (epidurals) or other
procedures, such as radiofrequency ablation, whereby the nerves are actually burned with electric current to prevent them from transmitting
pain signals. When those procedures don't work, the pain specialist or
clinic might refer the patient to a surgeon who, in all likelihood, would
suggest surgery because the medications and other techniques weren't
successful in relieving the pain. If a surgery was performed and judged a
"failure" because it didn't offer long-lasting pain reduction, the surgeon
might suggest more surgery or, just as likely, tell the patient that even
though the pain persisted, the surgery was technically a success and
therefore there was nothing more that could be done.

In essence, the message to the patient would be: "I did my job, so if
you're still in pain, you're just going to have to live with it," almost im-
plying, "It's your fault!" (That's exactly what happened to Loretta after
her fourth surgery.) A referral to a neurologist or rheumatologist might
come next. Or a psychiatrist, who might prescribe antidepressants and
more anti-anxiety medications. And on and on it goes.

At the time, back in 2006, I had almost twenty-five years of experience in addiction medicine. I was an expert at detoxing patients and
guiding them through the recovery process from the disease of addiction. But when it came to chronic pain, I felt horribly inadequate. Loretta was not an isolated case—a huge percentage of the patients I was
treating for opioid addiction, perhaps as many as 50 percent, were also
experiencing chronic pain. In fact, many had started using opioid drugs
because they were in pain, not because they wanted to "get high." What
was I going to do with these patients? How was I going to help them?

I knew at that moment that if I wanted to successfully care for
people who were dependent upon or addicted to opioids and who are
also living with chronic pain, I had to strip myself of those automatic
judgments, learn everything I could, and find creative and innovative

ways to approach the problem of chronic pain. I was already well equipped with a team of caring, highly skilled professionals adept at helping addicted patients by guiding them into long-term recovery. Adding chronic pain to the treatment plan would require that we rethink our approach and adjust our clinical services.

PASSED DOWN THE LINE

If you are a person in chronic pain, you will almost certainly know what I am talking about. You have been passed down the line and as the months and years wear on, assuming your doctors stick with you, they are likely to get more and more frustrated with their inability to relieve your pain. You might catch them rolling their eyes or checking their watch as you visit them. Trust me—they are unintentionally, even unconsciously, expressing their frustration and fear at their inability to help you. But of course that doesn't make you feel any better. As Diana, age seventy, says:

> I've lived with fibromyalgia for sixteen years. I know that all doctors are busy and I have yet to find a doctor who is interested in researching and finding out what is wrong with me. No doctor wants to even hear me say the word *pain*. That is a forbidden word now. My primary care doctor confessed he is afraid of me and my status as a chronic long-term pain patient. He is sending me to unsuspecting specialists. Having no safe, caring doctor in sixteen years has taken its toll on me, for sure.

Diana's complaints about her "doctor disasters" and the "You again?" attitude she feels every time she enters a doctor's office highlight a deeper problem. Doctors are, indeed, busy and often pressured to get patients in and out of the office as quickly as possible. It is rare for doctors to spend the time to research and find out the complexity of what is truly wrong with their patients—by research, I don't necessarily mean spending hours on the Internet (or, as we once did, in the library) but, rather, spending time with you, the patient, to uncover the multiple dimensions of your physical and emotional pain and really *listen* to you.

Acute pain is generally well managed and doctors are usually comfortable treating it, because the pain indicates tissue injury that can be treated effectively in most cases and, best of all, generally resolves within days to a few weeks. A child burns her hand on a hot stove . . . a woodworker slices off the tip of a finger with a skill saw . . . you twist your knee skiing . . . your appendicitis requires surgery. These are all repairable conditions, and doctors know what to do to treat the wound, reduce pain, and help you heal and move on with your life. Doctors also know that they have a willing and remarkable ally—your innate ability to heal. When an injury occurs, your body springs into action, initiating marvelously complex mechanisms to facilitate healing.

But chronic pain—lifelong pain that may ebb and flow depending on a variety of conditions but never wholly disappears—can be overwhelming to doctors. I am certain of one thing, which I have learned in recent years from teaching thousands of physicians about chronic pain and the inherent dangers of using opioid drugs for relief of chronic pain: Doctors get frustrated with their chronic pain patients because they are discouraged and disturbed by their inability to help you. We doctors get angry with you because we are annoyed with ourselves due to our own powerlessness. After many attempts, we may adopt what Diana calls a "get her outta here" attitude because you, the chronic pain patient, remind us that we do not have all the answers. With patients stacked up in the waiting room, that sense of powerlessness (and exasperation with our inability to do what we are supposed to do—heal the patient) leads to one of two solutions: write a prescription or admit we can't help and refer you to a specialist. These actions relieve us of responsibility and require only a few minutes, whereas taking time to really listen to a patient—witnessing the pain, probing the physical, mental, emotional, and spiritual depths of the problem—may take hours.

EMOTIONS DRIVE PAIN

A few months after Loretta was in treatment at the Las Vegas Recovery Center (LVRC), I attended a conference sponsored by the California Society of Addiction Medicine. One of the full-day workshops was "Pain and Addiction: Addressing the Tough Cases." That's where I met Barry Rosen, MD, and Jodie Trafton, PhD, two brilliant, sensitive, and extraordinarily talented individuals who have had a profound and lasting impact on my work.

From the first time I met Barry, I knew I wanted to be like him. Gentle, self-effacing, and sweet natured, Barry radiated concern, empathy, and, yes, love for his patients. He stood well over six feet tall (at least in my memory), with big bushy eyebrows, a receding hairline, and dark brown eyes that conveyed warmth and intelligence.

I loved watching him interact with patients. He would sit down next to them, often patting their hands or gently touching their shoulder as if to say, "I'm here, I'm listening; nothing is more important to me right now than you and this moment." Fear, anger, and hostility seemed to evaporate as they realized that he was not the "MD-eity" they had come to expect but, rather, a fellow human being who wanted nothing more than to help them and ease their concerns. Rarely had I seen a doctor interact with a patient in a way that conveyed such depth of caring and human connection.

Witnessing these interactions, I understood immediately why patients trusted him—why they loved him. He was so completely different from most of the physicians I had encountered in my life (including me at the time), who seemed always to be pressured by time and thus impatient, curt, and even rude as they delivered their diagnoses and medical advice in a stern and professional tone of voice, often finishing their patients' sentences for them, scribbling barely readable prescriptions, and ending the brief interview by looking at their watch with a weighty expression to indicate "time is up."

From watching Barry with his patients and working hard to model his unique, empathic style, I learned essential lessons that I use every day in my own work with people in chronic pain. From Jodie Trafton, who has had an equally profound influence on my life and my work, I learned what goes on inside our brain to drive us to think, behave, and emotionally respond in ways that cause us long-term harm. The basic principle here is that our brain is circuited to take shortcuts, even if the quicker route ends up not being in our best interest in the long run. For example, if you take an opioid medication, you get an immediate hit in your brain that is more instantaneous and powerful than the endorphin "high" generated by exercising. And exercise can be drudgery, with gains accumulating only with consistent effort and over time.

Furthermore, if you're in a lot of pain, exercise may actually make you feel worse temporarily. Exercise is thus the "longer" route and, when gauged in terms of instant relief, not necessarily the most "scenic" pathway. It makes sense that a brain that has become accustomed to the immediate reward and relief of opioids would choose that pathway. In contrast to the "no pain, no gain" rule of exercise, opioids offer the alternate route of "less pain, less gain."

Barely five feet tall (when she was seven or eight months pregnant, I remember fearing she would topple over), Jodie is brilliant, most evident in her descriptions of work in the research lab, where she has studied brain circuits and neurotransmitters involved in addiction and the behavioral consequences of neuroplastic changes, and on the lecture circuit, where she summarizes this elegant research for physicians like me. Although much of the information she discusses in her talks is hard to follow, I've been able to latch on to key pieces and a deepening understanding of the neurological underpinnings of habit formation and willpower. Jodie also describes how addictive drugs pharmacologically hijack the brain's reward system, causing dopamine neurons to fire vigorously, triggering huge rewards that in turn lead to craving for more drugs to experience more rewards.

In one of the first of a half-dozen lectures I heard Jodie give, she described an experiment that appeared in the *Journal of Neuroscience* in 2004 in which research subjects received an electric shock. If they pressed a button quickly enough, they were told, they could modify the intensity of the shock so that it was less painful. Subjects reported that pressing the button worked to reduce pain, and scientists confirmed through MRIs that there was less brain activity, indicating lower pain levels—and yet the button was not connected to anything. In other words, the subjects' expectation that they would have less pain if they quickly pushed the button, led to reduced signals in the pain-receiving areas of the midbrain and a decrease in their pain levels. As I listened to Jodie lecture, I got really excited, because it validated what I witness in my work with patients—if you "push the button" of believing good things will happen in treatment, knowing that you have some control over your situation, your pain lessens. The better the sense of control you have over your situation and the more you commit to the work needed to continue to reduce your pain, the greater the benefit of the treatment.

THE GIFT OF PAIN

Not long after I met Barry and Jodie, I picked up a copy of *The Gift of Pain* by Dr. Paul Brand and Philip Yancey.

A compassionate healer and consummate storyteller, Dr. Brand spent much of his life working in India with patients who had Hansen's disease, a bacterial infection more commonly known as leprosy. The prevailing medical theory held that leprosy itself caused grotesque disfigurements in untreated patients, whose noses sometimes shriveled away or who lost fingers and toes and would often go blind. From the work he did with patients in India, Dr. Brand arrived at a different theory: People with leprosy had disfigurements because the disease-causing bacteria destroyed the nerves that signaled pain. And without pain to guide them, they unwittingly put themselves in harm's way.

While researching his theory at a leprosarium in New Guinea, Dr. Brand observed a woman roasting yams over red-hot coals. One of the yams fell into the fire and as she tried to stab it with a stick, she drove it deeper into the blazing hot coals. She motioned to an old man sitting nearby, who shuffled over to the fire, reached into the coals with his bare hand, and rescued the yam. With no expression of pain whatsoever, he returned to his seat. Shocked and horrified, Dr. Brand immediately went to the old man's aid and examined his hand—it was covered with oozing blisters and scars. Although he eventually lost his hand, the old man displayed "an utter nonchalance toward self-destruction," in Brand's words, because he did not, could not, feel pain.

Pain, as unpleasant and even dreadful as it can be, serves a life-giving purpose by protecting us from hurting ourselves. In fact, it is precisely the unpleasantness of pain that warns us away from the cause of the pain, thus protecting our body from damage.

Yet prolonged pain can also become a destructive force. People with *chronic* pain can experience such interminable agony that they may begin to question the meaning and value of life itself. Some, tragically, feel like a mere shell of their former self and don't want to go on living. Thus in this modern age of believing that virtually all ills can be defeated with the right procedure or drug, we view chronic pain as the enemy to be defeated, a mysterious, unrelenting force that strips us of our strength and dignity, and a harsh reminder of our own limitations and powerlessness.

How, then, can there be "virtue" in chronic pain? With another story in the first chapter of *The Gift of Pain*, Dr. Brand recounts "the darkest night" of his life. After a week-long bout with influenza and an exhausting trip, Dr. Brand was suddenly, terrifyingly aware that part of his foot was numb.

> *I had no feeling in half my foot.* I sank back into a chair, my mind whirling. Perhaps it was an illusion. I closed my eyes and pressed against my heel with the tip of a ballpoint pen. Nothing. No sensation of touch whatsoever in the area around the heel.
>
> A *dread fear worse than any nausea seized my stomach*. Had it finally happened? Every leprosy worker recognizes insensitivity to pain as one of the disease's first symptoms. Had I just made the wretched leap from leprosy doctor to leprosy patient?

Dr. Brand knew all too well what to expect after working with hundreds of leprosy patients. "Ordinary pleasures in life would slip away," he wrote. "Petting a dog, running a hand across fine silk, holding a child—soon all sensations would feel alike: dead." He feared his career as a surgeon would end. What would happen to his work, his patients? Worst of all, he would need to shut himself off from his children, for children are most at risk of infection. Frightened and alone, he would join "the society of the accursed."

After a sleepless night, he woke up, jabbed his heel with a sewing needle, and immediately felt the sharpness of the point. With the pain came overwhelming waves of relief and joy. His heel, he realized, had been temporarily numb, most likely from sitting too long in one position. He could feel pain, there was no leprosy, he was free—and for the first time he understood at a deep, visceral level why leprosy victims look with envy upon those of us who feel pain. In this story, Dr. Brand also illuminates the emotions associated with chronic pain, especially fear and anxiety about the unknown, and he demonstrates negative projecting and catastrophization, which we will discuss later in the book.

Later in his career, Dr. Brand had the opportunity to work with rheumatoid arthritis patients, who begged him to relieve their pain with drugs. Some patients took such massive doses of steroids in an ill-fated attempt to relieve their pain that their bones gradually decalcified, growing soft, fragile, and vulnerable to injury.* One bedridden patient had taken so many steroids that "when she finally ventured from bed her foot bones crumbled like chalk." Reflecting on the nature, purpose, and meaning of chronic pain, Dr. Brand describes what he calls "the conundrum of pain."

"Why," Dr. Brand asked himself, "would our own minds inflict on us a state that we automatically choose against?"

PAIN'S PARADOX

Pain functions to protect us. When we are hurt or injured, the life-saving message we require to save us from further injury is: "Pay attention to me! *Now! Something is wrong!*" Pain is a warning sign, a red flag alerting us to danger, and its signals and symptoms serve to protect us from harm. Which makes perfect sense when we are talking about acute pain—but why does pain persist when it has accomplished its essential function, when its meaning and purpose have been fulfilled? This is what I see as pain's paradox: while pain is an exquisitely intricate and impossibly complicated system designed to protect us from harm, this system also can go haywire, lasting long after it has outlived its main purpose—that of warning us that something is wrong. People with chronic pain do not get the same relief that comes with the healing of a broken arm, a ruptured tendon, or a surgical incision. The pain

---

* In a prophetic footnote (*The Gift of Pain* was published in 1993, two years before Purdue Pharma introduced OxyContin to the world) Dr. Brand writes, "If we suppress the need for brain endorphins (the body's natural painkillers) by providing artificial substitutes, the brain may 'forget how' to produce the natural substances. Heroin addicts show the final result: an addict's brain demands more and more artificial substances because it can no longer satisfy the cravings of its own opiate receptor sites. Long-term heroin addicts sometimes develop a hypersensitivity to pain after they come off the drug. The slightest pressure of a sheet or clothing causes intense pain because the brain no longer manufactures the neurotransmitters that deal with such routine stimuli." We will explore the role of neurotransmitters, opioid receptor sites, and hypersensitivity to pain in the next chapter.

lingers even though it serves no purpose. This is what physicians call maladaptive pain—it sets up house (a distinctly unwelcome guest) in the pain center in our midbrain. And it never goes away.

Never? You might be tempted right now to toss this book in the nearest wastebasket. But please—*don't give up now or you'll miss the best part.* I am here to tell you there is a way out. You don't have to have a miserable life because of pain. You can learn how to manage your pain so that it no longer rules your life and your relationships.

FIVE FUNDAMENTAL LESSONS ABOUT CHRONIC PAIN

Throughout much of my career as a physician, I believed that pain was based in anatomical structural abnormalities or disease processes that damage the nerves locally within the tissue—a broken ankle, a surgical incision, back pain from a herniated disk, diabetic neuropathy, or neurological diseases, such as multiple sclerosis. I thought all kinds of pain were treatable with the right medication, procedural intervention, or operation. For many years I did not understand that the complex disorder of chronic pain is directly and intimately related to the organ system that's housed in our skull—the brain. Nor did I fully comprehend the fact that chronic pain is, in large part, driven by our thoughts and emotions.

I learned these lessons from the best teachers of all—my patients. If you are living with chronic pain, my hope is that these lessons will validate your experience and help you take the first steps toward achieving balance in your life. And if you are a medical professional, I hope they will help guide you in your interactions with your chronic pain patients.

Lesson #1: ALL PAIN IS REAL. Far too many of us (and I include myself, for I, too, live with chronic pain—more about that later) are chronically misunderstood. I've witnessed firsthand the high cost of having someone doubt the truth of my story, the reality of my pain. I've also been in the position of questioning the accuracy of another human being's assessment of their own pain, as I did with Loretta at the start of this chapter. I am now firmly convinced that this skepticism and disbelief impeded my ability to help.

When you tell your doctor that you have a high level of pain, what happens inside you when you notice the signs—the subtle looking away, the roll of the eyes, the gaze that drops, or some facial expression that you instantly recognize as doubt (or, worse, distaste)—that the person who is responsible for your care does not believe you? That doesn't feel very good, and it does not give you confidence that you are in the right place. Family members and friends may engage in the same doubting attitudes, which can strain relationships in both subtle and significant ways.

In a 2013 paper titled "A Narrative Review of the Impact of Disbelief in Chronic Pain" (published in the journal *Pain Management Nursing*) author Benjamin Newton and his colleagues discuss the feelings of rejection and isolation, along with the shame, humiliation, and self-doubt, experienced by individuals with chronic pain who are confronted with disbelief about their pain. The consequences of disbelief (often arising from the "invisibility" of chronic pain) are serious and profound, even to the point of affecting an individual's personal integrity and self-identity and leading to depression, guilt, anger, helplessness, and hopelessness. Newton and colleagues conclude:

> The invisibility of pain is possibly the central problem that sufferers face, and it is this aspect of pain that affects the identity of individuals. The lack of evidence to demonstrate the reality of the individual's experience may lead others to question the credibility of the patient. Such questioning can affect the sense of integrity that individuals wish to maintain.

Even with the most advanced tests and techniques that can pinpoint where we feel pain in the brain and body, the truth remains that your experience of pain is personal and unique. In other words, your pain is what you say it is. Doctors don't have a "Pain-o-Meter" that we can hook you up to so as to assess your pain level, nor do we have a blood test or X-ray that can detect or quantify your experience of pain. Although such research labs as Stanford are working on quantifying pain with the use of sophisticated functional MRI scans, at this point in time we do not have an objective way to measure pain in day-to-day practice.

What we do have are the totally subjective and rather inadequate and simplistic 0 to 10–point pain scales that are supposed to represent

Comparative Pain Scale

	0	No pain. Feeling perfectly normal.
Minor Does not interfere with most activities. Able to adapt to pain psychologically and with medication or devices such as cushions.	**1** Very Mild	Very light, barely noticeable pain, like a mosquito bite or a poison ivy itch. Most of the time you never think about the pain.
	2 Discomforting	Minor pain, like lightly pinching the fold of skin between the thumb and first finger with the other hand, using the fingernails, or an aching joint that is just noticeable but still in the background.
	3 Tolerable	Very noticeable pain, like an accidental cut, an injection or blood draw, or a blow to the face causing a bloody nose or black eye. The pain is not so strong that you can't get used to it and after a period of time, it goes away.
Moderate Interferes with many activities. Requires lifestyle changes but patient remains independent. Unable to adapt to pain.	**4** Distressing	Strong pain, like an abscessed tooth or an inflamed arthritic joint. So strong you notice the pain many times during the day and cannot completely adapt to it.
	5 Very Distressing	Strong, deep pain, such as chronic low back pain or spraining your ankle and then twisting it again. Not only do you notice the pain all the time, you are now so preoccupied with managing it that your normal lifestyle is curtailed.
	6 Intense	Strong, deep, piercing pain so intense it seems to partially dominate your senses, causing you to think somewhat unclearly. At this point you begin to have trouble focusing on your job or maintaining normal social relationships. Comparable to a ruptured ligament or tendon or an unrelenting migraine headache.

continues

continued

Severe Unable to engage in normal activities. Patient is disabled and unable to function independently.	**7** **Very Intense**	Pain so severe that it completely dominates your senses, causing you to think unclearly much of the time. At this point you are effectively disabled. Comparable to an unhealed fracture of the wrist or elbow that constantly throbs and aches.
	8 **Utterly Horrible**	Pain so intense you can no longer think clearly at all. If the pain has been present for a long time, you may experience severe personality changes. Suicide may be considered and may even be attempted. Comparable to a serious burn or untreated stomach ulcer.
	9 **Excruciating Unbearable**	Pain so intense you cannot tolerate it and can't picture life without painkillers or surgery, no matter what the side effects or risks. If drugs or surgery don't work, suicide is frequently considered. Comparable to late-stage cancer, childbirth, or a kidney stone.
	10 **Unimaginable Unspeakable**	Pain so intense you may lose consciousness. Most people have never experienced this level of pain. Those who have suffered a severe accident, such as a crushed hand, and lost consciousness as a result of the pain (rather than from blood loss) have experienced level 10.

Permission: The original Comparative Pain Scale was developed in 2002 by Jack Harich, a systems engineer at Georgia Tech. The scale has been revised for this book with his permission.

a numerical calibration of the pain experience. I've come to learn that because your pain is real, the number you assign to your pain level is not very helpful in and of itself. Here's what I mean by that: I recently worked with a patient who always reported a pain score of 10 out of 10. With great frustration and not a little fury, he told me that "the nurses don't believe me when I tell them my pain score. They don't like me, and I don't think you like me because I'm not getting any better." The distress he was feeling, evidenced by his furrowed brow, red face, clenched jaw, and tightly scrunched-up shoulders, clearly revealed how much it cost him to hold onto this assessment.

"Your 10 is your 10, Mitch," I responded. "I get that you are trying to convey that you hurt an awful lot, but it's hard for the nurses and your fellow patients to understand that you are always in the worst pain ever." I gave Mitch the comparative pain scale and asked him to apply those words to his pain level. It turns out that he was so used to reporting 10 out of 10 because that's the way he convinced doctors to prescribe more medication for him. And of course, his chronic bladder pain from interstitial cystitis was severe. There was no doubt about that.

"Well," Mitch said, after studying the chart for several minutes, "I guess it's not the worst pain I've ever had. So, it's an 8½—are you happy, Doc?"

We shared a laugh and Mitch's perception of his very real pain shifted by 15 percent right then and there.

Let's drop the debate about whether your pain is real—because it is. I encourage you to trust your own experience. And as we move forward you will see that when you stop feeling the need to prove how bad the pain is, it very well may lessen and lose some of its power over your life.

Lesson #2: EMOTIONS DRIVE THE EXPERIENCE OF PAIN. I often get a call from a physician or concerned family member that begins with this question: "I'm not sure whether this is real pain or emotional pain—which you do you think it is?" My answer is always yes—yes, it is real; and yes, it is emotional. After all, emotions are just as real as physical sensations.

Many of the people I see in treatment are medicating emotional pain that they perceive as physical pain. They feel anxious and their back starts to hurt, so they take a dose of medication. Remember Lesson #1—you are not making it up. And once you understand and internalize Lesson #2—emotions drive the experience of pain—you will see how "real" your pain is. Anxiety does cause you to hurt more. Fear causes you to hurt more. Anger causes you to hurt more. In my experience, chronic pain is about 20 percent sensory (physical) and the rest, the other 80 percent, is emotional. The key emotions that make pain worse are fear, anxiety, anger, guilt, grief, and helplessness. (See Chapter 3 for an in-depth discussion of these emotions.)

Believe me, I understand from my own personal experience with chronic pain that it may be difficult to wrap your mind around the fact that your emotions not only generate but also perpetuate your pain. But I encourage you to try this little exercise: Close your eyes and locate the places in your body where you hurt. Now focus in on the place that is bothering you most. For me, it's my lower back on the left side. As I close my eyes, I experience a tight sensation at the upper part of my butt with a burning and irritating sensation that travels down the outside of my left thigh. Immediately I feel frustrated. Actually, the emotion is more intense than frustration—I *hate* this pain. For the last decade it has been with me every moment of every minute of every hour of every day—and much like you, *I don't want it to be there!*

As I experience the emotions of irritation and exasperation, my muscles tighten up and the pain gets worse. Suddenly I'm afraid that I'm going to have a miserable day and night, because that's the story I have been telling myself for years whenever the pain flares up and threatens to negatively affect me. I won't be able to sleep and, damn it, I have a full day of patients to see tomorrow, in addition to a staff meeting and a paper to prepare for an upcoming conference. Now I'm angry and a tad bit resentful—why did this have to happen to me? All I did was lean over to pick up a stupid carry-on bag. One little twist twelve years ago and my whole life changed. With those thoughts my anxiety increases—*my whole life? Am I going to have to live with this pain for my whole life?* My heart starts beating a little faster, my head feels "fuzzy," and I'm having trouble concentrating.

My thoughts drift to my age. How much worse is this going to get when it's compounded by the predictable and unavoidable problems of growing older, aging bones, arthritis? Will I be able to tolerate it if it gets any worse? I can't and won't take opioids because I'm in long-term recovery and even if I could, I have learned too much about the dangers of these drugs to even approach that pathway. But my back is throbbing and the disturbing thoughts continue. Will I be able to survive this ever-worsening pain without drugs? Now my muscles are really tight and the pain is worse, jumping from a score of 3 to 5 or even 6 in just a few minutes.

And right about then I am able to catch myself and stop the cycle of emotionally driven pain. I take a deep breath and bring myself back to earth, to this moment, calming myself with what I know to be true—the burning, radiating pain from the bulging disk pressing on the nerves in my low back is only a small part of my overall experience of pain. That's the sensory experience and, yes, the pain is all too real. But most of my experience of pain—and virtually all my mental and emotional distress, my suffering—is related to my very human response of wanting to push away something that I don't like but can't avoid, being angry at myself for causing the injury in the first place, feeling a lot of fear about things that haven't happened and may never happen, and letting my thoughts carry me away into a future fantasy (misery) land of intolerable pain and decrepitude.

I can honestly say that this cycle of mental and emotional anguish captures the essence of my own experience as well as what I see, hear, and feel when I am with my patients. I have to tell you, however, that this is the lesson about which I get the most push back from patients who infer that by giving emotions such a powerful position in the experience of chronic pain, I am actually demeaning their experience of pain. Nothing could be farther from the truth. Your emotions are not imaginary constructs but *real* physiological events taking place in your brain that then trigger a cascade of consequences leading to *real* physical pain.

I hope I have made it clear that your pain *is* real—not just to you, but to me and many other doctors and health care practitioners who understand chronic pain. Emotions help drive your pain, but they do not in any way, shape, or form make it less real.

Lesson #3: OPIOIDS DON'T ALWAYS MAKE CHRONIC PAIN BETTER—in fact, they often make it worse. No scientific evidence exists to show that long-term (three months or longer) use of opioids effectively reduces chronic pain. I need to repeat that sentence to underscore its critical importance: Not one scientific study shows that opioids are effective for chronic pain if taken for more than three months. Steady use of opioids causes a multitude of serious side effects and, sometimes, life-threatening results. Furthermore, in far too many cases, opioids backfire and can actually cause more pain—the phenomenon known as opioid-induced hyperalgesia, which we will discuss in detail in the next chapter.

If you're not quite ready for this one, you're not alone. One of the hardest parts of my work is trying to explain to my patients that opioids are, in all likelihood, making their pain worse. Certainly for the acute pain of a broken leg or a kidney stone, or postoperatively, opioids are effective and appropriate as a short-term treatment over a finite time period. But with opioid use for chronic pain, increasing doses, increasing pain, decreased function, and inability to discontinue the drugs without significant withdrawal symptoms, lead inevitably to poor results. Of course, "poor" is an understatement when it comes to the ever-present realities of drug dependence, addiction, overdose, and death.

So—if you take opioids for an extended period of time (longer than three months), your body responds by creating more pain. Yes, that's right—your painkilling drugs are functioning as pain-creating drugs, increasing and exacerbating your pain. If you stop taking the drugs—and I know this is hard to fathom—your pain will lessen. Over the years I've treated hundreds of patients on very high doses of opioids, and with very few exceptions, pain levels decrease significantly when the drugs are discontinued.

It's amazing to me how many patients respond to that information with the words, "I kind of knew that, but I was afraid to believe it because then I'd have to give up my safety net." Others look at me as if I'm nuts, saying, "No way!" But what about you? Are you willing to consider the possibility that your drugs might be increasing your pain? Many of my patients offer two basic responses to that question. Perhaps these express your feelings as well?

Response #1: "When I take a pill, I know that there will be some small measure of decrease in my pain. Yes, the relief is short lived, but it is precisely that reliable decrease in pain, that experience of 'taking the edge off' that I've come to depend on."

Response #2: "How bad is my pain going to be when I stop? It only makes sense that the pain is going to be much, much worse, and it is already so terrible. How could I possibly bear it?"

I can only reassure you that (1) the short-lived relief you experience after taking your pills is not in any way, shape, or form worth the long-term escalation in your pain, and (2) you can bear it. You can bear it because, like thousands of other people living with chronic pain, you will have significantly less pain when the drugs are out of your system. And so the tough part is to take that leap of faith. You will need to believe me when I tell you that these drugs are not your best friend but in fact, may be your worst enemy.

Why should you trust me? What if I'm wrong? What if the pain gets worse? And my answer to these questions is: "You can always go back to this life that you've been living with the opioids." But if I'm right, your life will get better when the drugs are eliminated. In fact, your life may improve beyond your wildest dreams!

After a recent weekend working with family members, I was approached by Joe, a big burly midwesterner who I guessed was in his midsixties. Joe's wife had been in treatment for thirty-five days for chronic pain and addiction to OxyContin.

"I don't know how to thank you," he said, shifting from one foot to the other, clearly uncomfortable with the emotions that threatened to overwhelm him. On the verge of tears, he said in a choked-up voice, "I have my wife back. She has a sparkle in her eyes and a spring in her step. For the fifteen years she was using those damn pills, that sparkle, that spring were gone. She was gone. Now she's back."

Eliminating opioids from your life is not just about lowering your pain levels—it's about waking up and noticing that the sky is blue . . . getting the sparkle back in your eyes . . . reconnecting with the people who love you and who are suffering with you . . . and, to be frank, having a good bowel movement without a laxative (since opioids are constipating).

Lesson #4: FOCUS ON IMPROVING FUNCTION. With most chronic pain conditions, the goal of eliminating pain altogether is not realistic. Improvement of function, on the other hand—being able to engage in activities, interact in joyful ways with your family and friends, and be productive and active *despite the pain*—should be the preeminent concern for both you and your doctor.

If you don't focus your energies on improving your life rather than simply decreasing your pain, you are shortchanging yourself. If your doctors aren't asking about your function—in other words, "How far can you walk? How is your sleep? Are you participating in activities with your family? Are you awake when you want to be awake (or are you falling asleep in your soup at the dinner table)?"—then they are missing the purpose of appropriate pain treatment, which is to make you feel, act, and react *better*—to help you get out of bed, be awake and alert during the day, look around you with joy and even wonder, get a good night's sleep, and have your soup *in* you instead of *on* you.

I take a holistic approach to the treatment of illness. What are the appropriate goals of pain recovery? Are they simply to bring your pain score down from a 7 to a 5? I think not—I surely hope not. In fact, you will find that your pain score—the magnitude of your pain—is much less important in the long run than your overall engagement in life is. I see so many people admitted into treatment who are on high doses of painkillers, prescribed by well-meaning doctors and health-care practitioners, whose lives have essentially disappeared.

"I didn't exist," Ella, 56, said, describing the years she spent addicted to opioid medications prescribed for fibromyalgia and pain following two unsuccessful spinal surgeries. "My body moved through space, slowly and painfully, but the caring, energetic, creative person I used to be was gone, blotted out by the drugs. Everything that I used to be simply vanished without a trace."

If your doctors are treating you with the goal of taking your pain away, but you are actually feeling worse, incapable of leading an active and productive life, that is just not proper pain treatment. If you are not feeling better and you are less able to participate in life, where is the benefit of the treatment?

Lesson #5: EXPECTATIONS INFLUENCE OUTCOME. The answers to many of the problems that plague those of us who live with chronic pain lie in the power of our mind. Hundreds of scientific studies prove that our beliefs and predictions about the future—our expectations—have a profound impact on what happens next. Simply believing that a treatment will work often results in a positive outcome. Alternatively, if we have a "negative outcome expectation" of a specific treatment modality, we may have created a self-fulfilling prophecy. (The placebo effect, which we will discuss in Part 2, offers a compelling example of the power of expectations.)

The idea that your expectations—of success or failure—will have a profound impact on your physical and mental health may be difficult to accept. Like others who have extensively studied this phenomenon, however, I am convinced that most of us have tapped into a mere fraction of the true power of our minds. I think of yogis who can slow down their heart for minutes at a time, to the point that even a stethoscope can't detect a heartbeat. I think of people who walk again after their spinal cord has been "irreparably" injured or of severely brain-injured patients who return to a full and active life. Miracles happen every day. How can we explain them? Many of us shake our head and write them off to unbelievable, inexplicable phenomena that belong in Ripley's Believe It or Not! museums but could never happen to us.

I challenge you to suspend your disbelief and read this book with an open mind and heart. I promise that if you take that leap of faith into what may seem like the unknown and unlikely—if you commit yourself heart and soul to the concepts and strategies described in this book— you will experience a real and lasting transformation in your physical, emotional, mental, and spiritual health. Let me repeat—if you are open to possibilities, *miracles happen every day*.

An important note about discontinuing medications. Throughout this book, we'll talk about life without painkillers. Here is some information you absolutely need to know about discontinuing your medication:

Do not simply stop your medications. Over time, your body most likely has become accustomed to them and you may be physically dependent on them. Simply stopping these medications suddenly may be dangerous. You must consult a knowledgeable health-care provider or treatment center to supervise withdrawal from habit-forming medications, including opioids, sedatives, hypnotics, and alcohol.

TWO

BRAIN MATTERS
How Chronic Pain Changes the Brain

The most complicated three-pound
mass of matter in the known universe.

—JAY GIEDD, NEUROSCIENTIST

Two years ago, Paul arrived at Las Vegas Recovery Center from
the Deep South.

"I'm a Southern Baptist kid, sir," Paul proudly announced during
our intake interview. We both laughed. Although he was in his early
fifties and a physician, Paul did indeed look like a little kid with his
cherubic face and earnest expression—and even more so when he took
to wearing a red bandana as a headband when working out. If I needed
to describe him in a few words, they would be *unassuming, earnest, hum-
ble*, and even, perhaps, a little *goofy*.

I liked him immediately. His open-mindedness and willingness to
learn and engage in treatment were a breath of fresh air. He absorbed
information like a sponge, gratefully and good-naturedly accepting the
plan that the treatment team laid out for him.

"What's a doctor from the Deep South doing here in Las Vegas?" I
asked. I knew the outline of Paul's story—chronic, disabling neck pain;
spinal fusion surgery; increasing pain; addiction to Vicodin, Percodan,
OxyContin, morphine, and fentanyl. But I wanted to hear his version,
in part to get to know him and in part to assess his attitude about engaging in the tough work that lay ahead.

"Well, I'm in a lot of pain and I take a lot of drugs. I'm in trouble," he said matter-of-factly. "The medical board referred me to the Physician's Health Program and they sent me here. My license to practice medicine is on the line if I don't complete treatment and stay off the drugs."

Paul's personal experience with chronic pain began on a dove-hunting trip to South America with several friends. "We were constantly shooting; there were doves everywhere, to the left, to the right, in front and in back of us. I was turning around with my gun raised, swiveling and shooting all day. By the end of that week, my neck was aching and burning. I'd never experienced that kind of pain before.

"When I returned home," Paul continued, "the pain got steadily worse. When non-narcotic drugs stopped working, I decided to get a full workup, including X-rays, MRI, bone scans, and nerve conduction studies. The X-rays showed evidence of disk degeneration but no nerve compression. Based on these tests, my internist assumed I had arthritis in my neck. I remember thinking, "Man, I had no idea that arthritis was this painful."

Over the next several months and continuing for a few years, the pain increased from relatively mild but annoying to a constant aching and burning sensation. "At that point my internist referred me to a pain management specialist where I was injected with steroids, had nerve blocks, tried physical therapy and a TENS unit, topicals, neuropathics, and radiofrequency ablation (RFA) where they use radio waves to burn the offending nerves—the whole gamut. I had some improvement with RFA, physical therapy, heat, and massage, but only for a short period. Topamax and Neurontin, both anti-seizure medications, helped with the pain but I had terrible side effects. I could not make myself eat and lost a drastic amount of weight, and short-term memory loss became a significant problem as I struggled to remember routine doses of meds.

"My pain was discrete, describable, reproducible," Paul continued. "I knew if I twisted or turned a certain way, I'd get a sharp blast of pain. I also knew that when I was at home and able to get in a comfortable position and go to sleep, the pain would ease up and maybe even go away. But it always came back."

Opioid therapy worked for Paul, for a while, and although he had spent most of his life avoiding drugs, he wasn't too worried about taking narcotics for pain, because he wasn't what he considered to be a typical drug addict. "The big thing with drug addicts, I was taught in medical school, is craving—whenever I listened to patients describe their craving, it was like describing a love affair but with a drug."

Paul smiled and spread his hands out with a rueful expression. "Well, I didn't have that. I had pain relief, euphoria, energy, and an over-all sense of well-being—which was a potentially lethal combination of positive gain from opioids for a hard-working physician in pain—and no disadvantages at all, not even constipation. I got all the good stuff and none of the bad stuff."

Or so he thought at the time. As it turned out, eventually the drugs—Vicodin for the first five years, then over the next ten years new prescriptions and escalating doses of Percodan, OxyContin, morphine, and, finally, fentanyl—weren't strong enough to get rid of the pain.

"I kept thinking something is wrong; this is more than arthritis; the pain is too intense," Paul said. "The MRIs didn't show anything but degenerative disk disease. I was advised to avoid surgery, but I kept spiraling down, circling the drain. In November 2011 I was at the point where I just couldn't live with the pain any longer. I was desperate for help and could barely function, I was taking way too many drugs at way too high doses, and by this time I was experiencing serious side effects—sedation, nausea, and pain spikes that led me to self-medicate. Even then I wasn't too worried—I figured I was a doctor, I knew how to control things, and I wasn't having classic cravings. I surely wasn't going to get addicted. And, after all, if I was going to be of any help at all to my patients, I had to have relief from the unrelenting pain—it burned, sometimes it stabbed, it was hot, then it was cold, it moved from here to there, and it was always with me. I could not make it go away.

"Finally I asked my medical partner for help. He made me consult with a spinal neurosurgeon, who found the previously undiagnosed osteophyte, or bone spur, 'harpooning' a spinal nerve in my neck exactly where the pain was. Finally, I had a reason for the pain. But two weeks after a single-level spinal fusion and removal of the spur, a new agony took over—the pain that I had lived with for ten years was joined by what I call 'the dark passenger' of obsession. I became obsessed with the unrelenting pain, constantly gauging my pain level, trying to figure out where it would be in an hour or two, and most important, how could I make it stop. My obsessive thinking then led to the compulsive use of the pain meds.

"One night, I was trying to finish work at the hospital, clearly impaired from pushing the meds too far because of this all new intensity with the pain, when a colleague expressed his concerns in a nonjudgmental way. I was honest with him about how the pain had changed and was becoming uncontrollable no matter what I did or what meds I took. I knew that something was wrong but again the tests and X-rays showed the surgery was healing nicely. A week later I met with the hospital's Wellness Committee. I was instructed to take a three-month medical leave from working in the hospital so I could cut back on work and not be on call. I still continued to work in the office and slowing down definitely helped.

"I went back to my surgeon, who referred me to a pain specialist who talked about something called 'opioid-induced hyperalgesia,' where the painkillers get wrapped up in a continuous feedback loop in the brain's reward center and rather than ease the pain, they increase it. I had never heard of hyperalgesia nor had any of my previous treating physicians, but the more I listened, read, and learned, the more it made sense to me. It sure sounded like it fit my situation because the drugs just didn't work anymore and the pain was unbearable. The pain had also changed from being distinct and reproducible to being vague and shifting in nature and location. Nothing worked any longer to make it better.

"So, after the intervention and armed with this information, I decided to detox myself. I toughed it out for a month and went from a level 8 to a level 5 pain but I never went below a 5. With no other understanding of how to deal with chronic pain except to take drugs, I went back to the pain management specialist and he put me back on the drugs I was taking before—Ultram, a fentanyl patch, and Cymbalta. Giving me drugs was the only thing anyone treating me knew to do to try to help me. And the drugs did help to temporarily ease the pain.

"But I felt better than I looked, apparently, because the investigator for the State Board of Medical Licensure showed up. Somebody reported me after the impairment incident at the hospital, as my speech was slurred and my balance and gait were affected. Thank God, no one was hurt and that was the only work-related incident.

Paul came to LVRC for a five-day evaluation that quickly turned into three months of treatment for the dual diagnosis of pain and addiction. "I just sort of folded in on myself and said, 'Okay.' Because, I was done. Finished. Defeated.

"So, I did everything the treatment staff asked me to do. There I was, a redneck southern doctor in Vegas, doing yoga, acupuncture, Reiki, body scans, meditation, chiropractic medicine, free writing, all the techniques and strategies that I was asked to do, with the hope that it would get me out of the pain. Once I surrendered, it was no longer about my license but it was now about my life and my family. I had hope again that I could have a life without chronic suffering and I was willing to go to any length to get it. Even if it meant hanging out with a bunch of funny-talking people who lived in the middle of a desert and wouldn't know good food if they fell into it! I worked hard and learned all that I could about what had been happening to me and the process of recovery. It worked. When I left, I was a new man, drug-free and with a pain level that rarely rose above a 2. I got my hope back. I got my life back."

Remembering, Paul smiled. "I'm out over a year and I look back on that man who left treatment at eighty days and realize he was just taking the first steps on this recovery path. And I look ahead, with hope and faith, knowing I'm still a newcomer. It's all about acceptance. If you work the program, you will recover. Guaranteed. Work it and work it hard."

Every six months Paul visits LVRC as part of his monitoring plan with his state's Physician's Health Program. We give each other a big hug, embracing as old pals who have been on similar journeys. Paul's treatment is a great success story—he's a better doctor (he was recently elected president of his state's Medical Association) and a better husband and father, and he is living a much, much better life. His story highlights virtually every detail I hope to convey in this chapter about what happens inside our brain when we develop chronic pain, when we take opioid drugs for pain relief, and when we discontinue the drugs with medical help and commit ourselves to a program of recovery.

I will now try to convey the basics about the neurochemistry of pain and pain relief, knowing from my own experience that if you are living with chronic pain, you want to get to the facts as soon as possible. I am a strong believer that this information and knowledge will serve you in your recovery process.

So, here goes: Brain and Pain 101, condensed into Six Basic Points.

1. SOMETHING HURTS. Chronic pain typically begins with some kind of insult to the body. Perhaps an injury causes the initial acute pain—a broken bone, burn, or cut, for example. In some cases, the injury is so minor that it doesn't register as significant. In Dr. Paul's case, for example, the initial neck pain generated by twisting his neck from side to side seemed at first to be minor, even inconsequential. Sure, his neck hurt, but he didn't classify the pain as an "injury"—he certainly didn't expect it to control his life for the next fifteen years. Instead it was an annoyance, an inconvenience, a temporary "pain in the neck."

For others, the injury is more obvious. In a TED talk titled "The Mystery of Chronic Pain," pediatrician and anesthesiologist Elliot Krane told the story of Chandler, 16, who fell on her outstretched arm and sprained her wrist during dance practice. She went to the hospital, X-rays confirmed that her wrist was only sprained but not broken, the injury was treated, and she was released. But then something much more complex, even mysterious, happened. Three months after the initial injury, Chandler returned to the clinic. Her arm was discolored, almost purple, and cold to the touch. The pain, which had spread in one direction from her wrist to her fingertips and in the opposite direction from her wrist to her elbow and almost to her shoulder, was constant and severe. "The lightest touch of her arm," Dr. Krane explained, "caused excruciating, burning pain."

2. NERVES REACT. For Chandler, for Paul, and for so many others, the initial, acute injury was only the beginning of a long, arduous, and confounding journey. For some reason and at some point in time—and no one knows exactly why or when—Chandler's nervous system overreacted. The nerves in her hand sent electrical impulses traveling as fast as 250 mph to her spinal cord, where a second set of nerves speedily transferred the pain signals up to her brain.

We're not talking about a simple relay race with a clean handoff from one nerve to another. It's much more complicated than that. When you are injured, thousands of nerves get into the race, spilling out their communication satellites (neurotransmitters) in all directions, up, down, in, out, around, about, and sideways to activate tens of thousands of nearby cells. Glial cells, in particular, play a central role in the regulation, intensification, and potential distortion of the sensory experience of pain. Once triggered, the cells' DNA starts mass-producing proteins, which interact with nearby nerves, which then release their neurotransmitters, which activate more cells, which produce more proteins, which interact with distant nerves and on and on it goes.

So far so good: The brain is alerted and can institute necessary protective actions—don't move or put pressure on the injured limb, wash and bandage the wound, seek medical attention for unrelenting discomfort—all of which serve to protect damaged tissue from further injury.

3. POSITIVE AND NEGATIVE FEEDBACK LOOPS.
In life, in general, we all need and want feedback—responses, comments, advice—so as to adapt, change, and grow. Feedback can be damaging, even destructive, however, when it involves disapproval, condemnation, or blame—and yet even when we are severely criticized or rebuked, we can learn from the situation, restore our state of balance, and move forward.

Your body is constantly and instantaneously making adjustments based on internal and external input. Its ability to self-regulate and self-organize depends upon feedback—for example, when your body temperature goes down, you shiver and when it rises, you sweat. These stress responses and regulatory processes cycle continuously, involuntarily, and subconsciously through your nervous, endocrine, immune, and other body systems to restore you to a state of internal balance.

Suppose you are in a car accident and although you have no major injuries, the air bag deployed, causing deep bruising to your chest and ribs. When the medic arrives and checks your vital signs, your blood pressure has spiked to 160 over 90 (it's usually in the 110/70 range). When your friend arrives at the scene and your stress and anxiety levels decrease as the medics reassure you that your injuries are minor and not life-threatening, your blood pressure also decreases.

You've just experienced a positive and a negative feedback loop. Your blood pressure "spiked," sending blood to all your vital organs in response to an emergency situation. That's an adrenaline-based, sympathetic nervous system "positive" reaction that allows your body to initiate emergency responses. When the traumatic situation resolves, your blood pressure returns to normal—that's "negative" feedback, which stabilizes the body's systems and returns the blood pressure and other vital signs to normal. Because we're dealing with a car accident in this example, imagine the positive feedback loop as pushing the gas pedal to the floor and the negative one as the process of braking and decelerating.

In some cases, however, the stress of the event keeps the positive loop in motion (imagine the engine revving), further accelerating the stress response so that your blood pressure stays elevated (hypertension). In one study of sixty patients with elevated blood pressure following an accident, fourteen people—nearly 25 percent—continued to have elevated blood pressure and received ongoing treatment for hypertension from their physicians. In these cases, the positive feedback system, which is necessary for emergent responding to a threat or danger, had gone awry, disrupting normal processes and leading to system malfunction. In essence, the "off" switch or "all clear" signal—the brakes—stopped working, with potentially destructive consequences.

This is what happened to Chandler after she fell and sprained her wrist—her positive feedback kept cycling while her negative feedback system failed to kick in. As Dr. Krane explains in his TED talk, "It's almost as if somebody came into your home and rewired your walls so that the next time you turned on the light switch, the toilet flushed three doors down, or your dishwasher went on, or your computer monitor turned off." If that happened in your home, you would probably be a little freaked out and call an electrician or plumber, or perhaps you'd try to fix the problem yourself. But this is all happening in your body without your conscious awareness and outside your control. When billions of cells are responding and releasing chemical and electrical signals, those inconceivably complex connections can overheat and become hyperstimulated. To make matters worse, a phenomenon called windup may occur, in which repeated stimulation of nerve fibers increases the spinal cord's electrical responses; this, in turn, intensifies your perception of pain. Your nerves are wound up into tighter and tighter coils that transmit signals of increasingly intense, constant pain.

While researchers are still developing their knowledge about the precise neuroanatomical mechanisms underlying chronic pain, recent studies suggest that a reverberating positive feedback loop is established in the brain and central nervous system, leading to hypersensitive pain pathways. While it's strange to think of a "positive" loop leading to such negative consequences, researchers are quick to point out that these loops are "inherently dangerous," for the "intrinsic 'turn-off' mechanism" either is not present or stops working. As the pain pathways become deeply entrenched, the brain adapts through structural changes that then impact and change the way your brain works. Chronic pain, in other words, reorganizes and restructures the brain. I want to restate this conclusion for it is truly astonishing: *Chronic pain is capable of altering the structure and the function of your brain.*

Researchers at the National Center for Complementary and Alternative Medicine (NCCAM) at the National Institutes of Health offer this synopsis of recent scientific studies:

> Chronic pain affects the anatomy of the brain and impairs certain nerve pathways . . . The evidence has been building that chronic pain can alter the functioning and anatomical integrity of various brain regions. This can lead, for example, to accelerated loss of gray matter, increased sensitivity to pain signals, reduced ability of the brain to release its own painkillers, emotional changes (such as anxiety disorders and depression), and cognitive deficits.

The good news, as reported by these researchers, is that mind and body approaches (meditation and yoga, for example) may have protective effects that help reverse these "chronic-pain-associated brain changes." These are among the approaches I will discuss in detail in Part 2.

4. PAIN BECOMES ITS OWN DISEASE. When acute pain progresses to chronic pain, pain itself becomes a disease. This progression is known as the chronification of pain. We still don't know exactly why it happens in certain people. What we do know is that brain activity shifts in the transition to chronic pain and that this shift may involve irreversible biologic factors, including an increase in the "excitability" of neurons within the central nervous system. This increased sensitivity is called central sensitization. It's as if the volume knobs in the pain-receiving and pain-perceiving parts of the brain are turned up several notches. Thus, some of us—perhaps one of every ten people—are "wired" to feel more pain than are others, due to pathological (abnormal) changes in brain structure and function.

Chronic pain becomes its own disease. Pain is no longer a symptom reflecting the body's protective response to an unpleasant or harmful stimulus, but a true physiological disease process resulting from neuroplasticity—the brain's ability to change its structure and function, which, in the case of chronic pain, leads to an increase in the intensity of experienced pain. Brain cells become sensitized to pain impulses and may overreact to the point that even a mere touch can cause excruciating pain. I had one patient who couldn't sleep because even the lightest touch of a bedsheet on her skin was painful; she rigged a metal bar on her bed so the sheet would still cover her but not touch her skin. Imagine her dismay when someone tried to hug her. And try to imagine how isolated she felt when even a gentle, sensitive touch made her cry out in pain.

Remember that all pain is real: it is critical to understand that being more sensitive to pain does not mean that you are making up, exaggerating, or imagining your pain. (Unfortunately, that knowledge doesn't always shield us from the judgments of others—or of ourselves.) Ellen, who couldn't bear the touch of a bedsheet, was not being a "crybaby." Gregory wasn't a "wuss" simply because he winced when someone gave him a strong handshake. Madelyn wasn't weak because she groaned every time she moved her shoulder. Walter wasn't a wimp because his knee hurt every time he stood up. Each of their experiences involved significant pain.

Real pain. In people with chronic pain, what would normally be a 0 to 3 response on a 10-point pain scale gets ramped up so that the pain score rarely falls below a 5 and often ranges between 8 and 9. Why this happens remains somewhat of a mystery, although researchers and pain medicine specialists are piecing together sections of this multitrillion-piece jigsaw puzzle. One part of this puzzle relates to variants of an enzyme called Catechol-O-methyltransferase (COMT) that metabolizes dopamine. (Often called the "pleasure" molecule, dopamine helps control the brain's reward and pleasure centers. Dopamine is also involved in motivating us to avoid unpleasant experiences.)

With certain variations in this enzyme (let's call this type A), sensations of pain become magnified. People with this variant tend to complain bitterly when touched lightly anywhere on their body. They feel more pain than do type B folks, who are bothered very little, if at all, by the same light touch. In short, type A people are physiologically circuited differently. These neurological changes may be genetically transmitted or they may result from an earlier traumatic experience—or, most likely, both. People who have experienced trauma in their lives—physical, sexual, or emotional—later develop different variants of COMT and, as a result, have lower pain thresholds. In other words, it takes less to make them hurt and when they feel pain, they hurt more.

Some symptoms of chronic pain that you may experience include allodynia and hyperalgesia. These two commonly used terms in pain medicine illustrate the complexity of this exaggerated or maladaptive pain response.

- **Allodynia:** Many of us know what it feels like to put on a shirt when we have a bad sunburn. Just the feeling of cloth touching skin is enough to make us wince and moan in pain. Allodynia is what happens when there is no sunburn—a painful response to a mild, normally harmless stimulus. Through an as-yet-unknown process, changes in the dorsal horn of the spinal cord (a common gathering place for nerve fibers where they connect with other neurons and continue their journey up to the brain) allow innocuous sensory information to get past the usual checkpoints that block access to the nociceptive (pain-sensing) system. Somehow these mild, harmless signals find their way around or through these security gates to activate nerve cell endings called nociceptors, which sense and respond by transmitting pain signals to the brain.

  Researchers are developing more precise knowledge about what happens in the dorsal horn, but for now we'll have to be content with the knowledge that in many people with chronic pain, the messaging system gets screwed up and information that normally would not gain access to the nociceptor system stuns the security guards, rams through the gate, and causes nerve cells to fire, signaling pain when there should be none.

- **Hyperalgesia:** Like allodynia, hyperalgesia is a sign of an amplified pain response. But unlike allodynia, where the stimulus is innocuous, with hyperalgesia the alarm signal is painful or noxious and your response to that signal is exaggerated. The noxious stimulus activates pain receptors in the periphery that then send the signal onto the spinal cord. Hyperalgesia involves an amplification of the pain signal. This amplification can occur in the periphery, where the tissue is sensitized by an irritant, by inflammation, or by disease; in the spinal cord; or in both locations. There are some cases where the amplification is thought to occur in higher brain centers as well. This can happen, for instance, after a stroke.

A good number of people reading this book will be familiar with hyperalgesia. That is because opioids cause hyperalgesia. Martin, for example, was a writer who had used opioids for fifteen years, ever since his wrist and elbow were injured in a car accident. In the intervening years he had developed, in his words, "total body pain." When I met him, he was taking both long-acting and short-acting morphine in very high doses (more than 400 mg total per day). Within a week of being detoxed from his opioid medications, much to his surprise and delight, the elbow and wrist pain dropped from a 7 on the pain scale to a 2, and the all-over body pain had totally disappeared. He was walking proof of the increased pain caused by opioids, which was relieved when the opioids were out of his system.

The pain you experience with hyperalgesia does not mean that your tissues are damaged but, rather, that your brain interprets the sensory signals from the painful stimulus as a threat and creates a pain impulse. This could be because your natural pain-relieving pathways are not working as they should be—or that your pain pathways are superactivated; that is, hyped up and on high alert. Your internal pain volume knob is turned up. The leap from 2 to 8 on the pain scale does not mean you're imagining the pain—the pain is real and it is being processed in your brain as potentially damaging or threatening, even though, in reality, it is not.

5. OPIOID-INDUCED HYPERALGESIA (also known as paradoxical hyperalgesia). "I'd never heard of hyperalgesia until my last pain doctor mentioned it," Paul told me during our initial interview at Las Vegas Recovery Center. "I still don't understand it. I just can't wrap my arms around the idea."

I explained to him, as I explain (usually more than once) to every patient who enters treatment with a dependence on or addiction to opioid drugs, that hyperalgesia can be endogenous—generated by an oversensitive, hyperactive nervous system—or it can be exogenous—induced by the drugs we take in an effort to relieve pain. Paul, like most patients, was struck by the paradox.

"So, you're telling me the drugs I take to reduce my pain have actually been making my pain worse?" he said.

"That's exactly what I'm telling you and anyone on opioids who will listen!" I responded with excitement.

I wasn't at all surprised by Paul's question. Only in the last ten to fifteen years have researchers confirmed that opioid drugs can cause central sensitization, a long-lasting condition or state of the nervous system that manifests in a heightened sensitivity to pain. In a 2003 article titled "Opioid Therapy for Chronic Pain," published in the *New England Journal of Medicine*, researchers Jane Ballantyne and Jianren Mao concluded: "Whereas it was previously thought that unlimited dose escalation was at least safe, evidence now suggests that prolonged, high-dose opioid therapy may be neither safe nor effective." This research evidence is only recently filtering down into public consciousness (and doctors' offices) as we learn that not only do opioid drugs stop working effectively to dull pain, but over time they actually start feeding and nourishing the pain—which often leads to taking higher and higher doses (more and/or stronger pills) to get any pain relief at all.

If opioids are causing more rather than less pain—in other words, they are backfiring—you might be wondering, as Paul did: "If I stop the opioids, will my pain levels decrease?" The happy answer is yes. For most patients I treat, pain levels go down, sometimes precipitously, when they stop taking opioid drugs. For you, it should be no different.

6. NEUROPLASTICITY. Your brain is constantly changing—even as you read this paragraph and commit bits and pieces to memory, you are rewiring your brain, laying down new track on the brain's railways. I recently came across this fascinating statement in John Medina's book *Brain Rules*: "A great deal of the brain is hard-wired *not* to be hard-wired. Like a beautiful, rigorously trained ballerina, we are hard-wired to be flexible." Our brain, in other words, is *always* adapting. With every new experience, thought, sensation, or life event, it is capable of creating new connections and altering existing pathways to adjust to changing circumstances, make room for additional information, and create new (or revise existing) memories. Neuroplasticity is the ability of our brain to establish fresh pathways consisting of millions of nerve cells with trillions of connections (approximately one thousand per nerve cell). The more a particular pathway within the circuit is activated—the more you play tennis, practice a musical instrument, sing a favorite song (the possibilities are endless)—the stronger the pathway becomes.

I recently heard a story about a school administrator who was in charge of determining where the sidewalks should go at a new school. He suggested waiting a bit—he wanted to see where the students walked to get from one class to another. When the grass was worn down along certain well-trodden pathways, he said, "That's where we should put the sidewalks." The brain can be said to perform a similar action—when a pathway is well traveled, the brain cements it over to make it easier to traverse.

Pain can be caused—and intensified—by these oft-used pathways. Even in the absence of an injury, when there is no broken bone, no infection, no tumor—no good reason for the pain—those neural sidewalks and superhighways can spark the nerves to fire pain signals again and again, in effect creating a self-sustaining circuit. Well-traveled pathways are very difficult, but thankfully, not impossible, to unlearn.

THE ROLE OF MEMORY

Memory plays a significant role in the experience of chronic pain. When we recall previous experiences from memory, the actual act of remembering assigns significance and meaning to current life events. In effect, when I feel discomfort in my low back, it taps into the memories of previous episodes of pain and what happened to cause that pain. Along with the pain I feel frustration. And sometimes, anger. "I've got lots of work to do and this is going to slow me down, just like the last time my back flared up," I say to myself.

Maybe when you remember an argument with your teenage son or daughter, you suddenly feel a headache coming on. "This one's going to be a doozy," you prophesize, "just like the last one I had when we argued." Or maybe you're playing golf and your partner calls out, "Good shot!" when you know it's a lousy shot (you end up in a sand trap). As you walk toward your ball, you remember the time you wrenched your shoulder trying to get out of a sand trap, and suddenly your shoulder starts throbbing. Sure enough, you bury the ball deeper into the sand, sending shooting pain from your shoulder all the way to your wrist.

The pain is still there the next day—in fact, it's worse. Crap. You feel guilty for being angry and not being able to shake it. And you remember other times in your life when anger got the best of you. Why can't you just let things go? The emotions intensify. Your shoulder is aching so badly. Three days, four days, and the pain is worse, throbbing and burning, a constant, nagging discomfort. Maybe something is really wrong. Did you do something to damage your rotator cuff? Maybe you need surgery. Suddenly an old memory returns and the details are vivid, almost as if you can see yourself in the green Plymouth forty years ago, stopped on a busy street to take a left-hand turn (you had your blinker on) and some old guy in a pickup truck rammed right into the back of your car. You flew forward and then backward with such force (no seatbelts back then) that the front-row seat was unhinged. Remembering, you wince and reach up to massage your sore shoulder. A week later the pain, now familiar, is worse than ever. What the heck is going on?

Your inflamed nerves have a memory and when you feel a twinge of pain, your emotions flare up and activate specific memories lodged in your hippocampus. Other memories join in. What began as a fine, easily erasable pencil mark in your neurocircuitry is now inked in. The pain continues, the memories are embedded and eventually outlined with permanent marker. The pain gets worse and it doesn't take long for the cement team to come in and pour concrete over the neural pathways. You're in chronic pain. Sure, it may ebb and flow, but it never goes away.

My friend David Hanscom, MD, author of *Back in Control*, offers a memorable explanation of the role of memory in the evolution of chronic pain:

> If you're one of the unfortunate people who experience pain longer than a couple of months, your pain may evolve into a neurological problem. When the nervous system is barraged day after day with pain impulses, many changes occur within the brain itself.
>
> As the brain's pain centers remain active they send out signals that alter the body's chemistry. The repetition of the pain impulses and resultant alteration in body chemistry causes you to become

sensitized to these signals. Eventually, the central nervous system "memorizes" the pain.

Memories, so useful and necessary to being human, play a major role in the evolution of chronic pain. Memories from many years ago—or just yesterday—connect to present-day experiences and your pain intensifies. Your emotional responses to the pain ensure that these memories will become firmly entrenched and therefore easily remembered, triggering even more pain.

EDDIE'S STORY

Eddie was an angry man. Fifty-four years old and a midlevel executive, he had been forced into retirement after working for the same large corporation for twenty-five years. Within minutes of walking into my office and settling himself into a chair, Eddie launched into an attack on his boss.

"He never liked me, he was always on my tail about something," Eddie said bitterly. "Just a few weeks before I lost my job, he hired some young guy, fresh out of business school for three quarters of my salary. I knew that young punk was hired as my replacement, but what could I do about it?"

As I sat at my desk during the intake interview, I was struck by the dullness of Eddie's eyes and the tight set of his jaw. He seemed depressed and angry. Despite all the drugs he was taking—high doses (120 mg) of methadone in addition to four or five 10 mg Percocets daily—he was strung tight. An old memory suddenly flashed through my mind. I was fifteen, tuning my guitar when, with one final rotation of the wing nut, the string broke. It occurred to me that was all it would take to make Eddie snap. I really wanted to avoid that one final twist.

"Tell me what brings you here, Eddie," I said, keeping my tone level and calm.

"My wife forced me to come. She found this place," he said. "She threatened to leave me if I didn't get off these damn drugs."

"Tell me about how the pain started," I said. We'd have time to talk about his family problems later.

"Well, okay," he grumbled, clearly reluctant to set his resentments aside. "About two years ago, I was cleaning out my office and lifted a heavy box of books. I felt this sudden white-hot pain radiating down my arm. I knew I'd done something bad but I thought it was in my shoulder. Later I found out I had ruptured a disk in my neck."

I am always amazed by stories like this, when life changes in an instant. I usually see patients months or years after their first experience with chronic pain, but when we travel backward to the moment when the disk ruptured or the headaches started, it seems there is almost an instantaneous shift from "no pain" to "lifelong pain." Everything changes just like that, in a moment, and for many of us nothing will ever be the same again.

I asked Eddie questions about his childhood and upbringing, as I always do. The memories of a traumatic event or a dysfunctional family life stay with us and can feed into the cycle of chronic pain. He offered short, guarded answers to my questions ("Why do we have to root around in the past?" he asked at one point). I learned that his dad was a plumber who worked fourteen hour days and "drank like a fish," while his mother worked equally long days as a waitress, leaving Eddie to care for his two younger sisters. As a child he found it difficult to make friends. "I didn't want anyone to see my dad drunk and he was always drunk," he told me.

Decades later, he was still filled with resentment, but I also picked up on his profound sadness and grief. Those emotions were pushed away quickly, however, as Eddie clearly wanted to stay with the anger that was familiar and made him feel strong, rather than with the sense of rejection, which left him feeling defeated and weak.

His tone became belligerent when he talked about his teenage years. "I didn't drink or use drugs, if that's what you're thinking," he said, almost spitting out the words at me. "I wasn't going to be an alcoholic loser like my dad. No way."

As Eddie's story unfolded over the next week, it seemed that his life experiences had gone from bad to worse. A difficult childhood, a loner with few friends, getting stuck in a boring job with a boss he hated, enduring the constant "nagging" from his wife and the arguments from his "ungrateful" kids, and then the injury and its aftermath—the ruptured disk, surgery, and the frustration and agony of chronic pain that seemed to intensify with each passing day. He took more and more pills for the pain ("The damn things stopped working after a while"). He lost his job and retained a "useless" lawyer who filed a claim for wrongful termination and helped Eddie file for disability benefits. His wife of thirty years fretted about finances and they argued constantly about his exorbitant medical and pharmacy bills. When his son accused him of exaggerating his pain to get out of looking for work, Eddie refused to have anything more to do with him.

"How dare he say that I was faking my pain," Eddie said, his face turning red. "That ungrateful little SOB."

But it was Eddie's childhood that kept coming up in our conversations. On our third day together, Eddie opened up about his abusive father who "never gave a damn about me or anything I did." Eddie never felt safe in his home but was always on alert, always on guard.

"One night my father got rip-roaring drunk and told me I was the cause of all his problems, that if it weren't for me, he'd have a different life and be a happy man." Eddie took a deep breath. "I was twelve. How the hell is a twelve-year-old supposed to handle that?"

Up until that moment, Eddie stoically recounted these painful encounters with his father. He looked at me for understanding, and I nodded my head, silently witnessing his pain. A moment passed and then his grief, shame, and sense of helplessness overwhelmed him and he started to cry. Tears ran down his cheeks and within seconds he was sobbing uncontrollably, bent forward in the chair, his head in his hands.

After a few seconds, I reached over and passed Eddie the box of Kleenex. Eddie blew his nose and then fixed me with a look full of rage—even hatred. I recognized that look from previous sessions with Eddie and also from dozens of encounters with other patients. Without having to say a word, the expression on Eddie's face screamed out at me, "You're making me feel miserable—how dare you disrupt my equilibrium?" A moment passed, after which Eddie sat back, dabbed (hard) at his eyes, clenched his jaw and stood up.

"I have to go now." And with sudden fury he shoved his chair back and stomped out of my office.

■ ■ ■

Although I am not a psychiatrist, I've studied enough counseling techniques and worked with enough patients in deep emotional pain to know that when the jaw tightens, the eyes flash rage, and the tears start to flow, some deeply guarded emotion might be making its way to the surface. (Note the word *might*—when working with emotions, it is always a good idea for me to leave room for other possibilities and allow my patient to correct any wrong assumptions.)

When Eddie broke down in front of me, he seemed to revert into that frightened, hurt little boy who on some level and for multiple reasons had never taken the opportunity to confront the sense of loss and loneliness that pervaded his childhood. As a young adult, Eddie left the past behind, or so he thought, swearing off all drugs, succeeding in college, marrying his high school sweetheart, raising two children, and vowing that he would never, ever be like his dad. And for years, he kept his promise to himself—he didn't drink or act out like his dad. But along the way Eddie had internalized so much rage that it had settled deep into his heart, his gut, his soul—and eventually, after the injury, in his spine.

Without his awareness and despite his best efforts, he had become bitter, angry, resentful, and depressed—just like his father. When he injured his neck, he had to deal not just with the pain but also with the fear that he would lose his job and become a "deadbeat" just like his dad. His deepest fear (although he was loath to admit it) was related to his dependence on opioids, for he was terrified that he might become addicted to drugs in the same way his father had become addicted to alcohol. Those fears, based on memories of his painful past, pervaded his present-day experience. His boss reminded him of his abusive father. When he played racquetball at the Y, before his injury, he was flooded with memories of his father, who would intentionally drill him in the back with the ball if he got in his way. When he argued with his wife or children, he felt as if he were looking in a mirror and seeing the very image of his father.

These memories and their attendant emotions greatly intensified his pain. Once again, I was witnessing in real life how our emotions can trigger and drive pain. Emotions, as we will explore in greater detail in the next chapter, loom large in our experience of pain.

THREE

EMOTIONS DRIVE PAIN

Painful Experiences
Are Emotional Experiences

As pain becomes chronic, the sensory components become less important and the emotional and behavioral components tend to take on more importance . . . Having pain is a strong emotional experience. It will reshape your behavior. It will reshape how you interact with the world. And that in itself means your brain is going to respond differently over time.

—JODIE ANN TRAFTON, PHD, RESEARCH HEALTH SCIENCE SPECIALIST, STANFORD UNIVERSITY

Over the next two weeks in treatment, Eddie's anger ebbed and flowed. He moved into "stoic" mode, accepting without complaint all the tools and strategies the staff offered him—group and individual therapy, free-writing, yoga, meditation, acupuncture (you will learn more about these in Part 2)—but he kept his emotions stuffed deep inside. Counselors reported that he would just sit passively in their groups, respectfully listening to other patients' stories but unwilling to share his own story. In our sessions together, he told me he couldn't do physical therapy because it hurt too much. In a dispassionate tone of voice, he reported that he was having heart palpitations and panic attacks.

His pain wasn't getting any better—it was still 8 out of 10—but in our sessions he attached no emotion whatsoever to the high pain scores. He was unable or unwilling to see the connection between his pain and his emotions. Having broken down in my office once, he was damned if he was going to do it again.

"Life just is what it is," he said, "and I really don't have anything else to say."

So, we had "the talk," one I've had with hundreds of patients in chronic pain.

"Look, Eddie," I said in his third week of treatment, "you know more about yourself than I do, but I know more about chronic pain than you do and here's what I know. Until and unless you deal with these emotions, you will not get better."

His response was somewhat predictable. He got red in the face and his hands clenched the sides of his chair so tightly that his knuckles turned white. "You're telling me I'll never get better! Why should I stay here, then? I should just go home right now!"

"No, Eddie," I said, "I'm telling you that if you keep your emotions locked up inside you, you may never find relief from your pain."

"How dare you suggest that emotions have anything to do with my pain?" he yelled at me. "Have you even looked at my MRI? Have you seen the scars from my surgery? You call yourself a doctor? What right do you have to speak to me about my emotions? You're not my shrink!"

I quickly realized that I had hit a nerve. In fact, I'd stirred up a whole tangle of nerves. "Hurt people hurt people," I repeated over and over again in my mind and the wisdom of those four simple words settled me, as they so often do.

Suddenly he stood up. "You're nuts! You don't understand me and you can't help me." And once again he stomped out of my office. This was becoming a pattern.

Eddie showed up in my office the next morning, his emotions again tightly under wraps, and announced that he was packing his belongings and leaving the program. He'd been thinking about what I had said and he had convinced himself that this program was not for him. With relative calm, he explained why. We were asking him to do things that he did not want to do and that he didn't think would help him. And, he added, "it's just too hard."

I pulled one last card out of my doctor deck. "Eddie, even though you think I am full of bull, I want you to give us another week to work with you," I said. "What do you have to lose if I'm wrong? You can go back to your old life. But what do you have to gain if I am right? Are you willing to do that?"

Eddie opened his mouth to argue with me and then closed it. As if in slow motion, he sat down in the chair, shoulders slumped, head bowed. After a few moments, I gently invited him to take a breath and open his fists. He looked down with surprise at his clenched hands as if noticing them for the first time. With obvious effort, he spread his fingers out straight and then let his open hands rest on his knees.

I took a deep breath and exhaled slowly. He did the same, mirroring me, as he stared down at his hands, clenching his fists and then opening them again. The synchronicity of the moment was powerful. When he finally looked up at me, he had a pleading look in his eyes. He began to speak softly, with deep sincerity, about how afraid he was of revealing emotions that he had sealed off for so long. But for the first time he didn't discount the fact that opening up and dealing with these emotions might be helpful for him. He expressed sadness and fear, rather than anger and bitterness.

I believe that was the moment when Eddie finally "surrendered" and the real healing began. When he gave in and stopped fighting, he began to change. Over the next few weeks, his pain dropped from a steady 8 to a 6 and then a 4. Remarkably and courageously he accepted the fact that anger was no longer working for him. The softer he got, the stronger he got—that paradoxical shift that occurs when we stop fighting the truth and let go of our efforts to control that which we cannot control.

Two years later Eddie remains free of drugs. Not so long ago, his wife called to let me know that his pain levels are manageable without drugs, his anger is also under control, he is much easier to live with, and he has made peace with his children. "He still keeps those emotions of his tightly controlled," she added and I could hear the smile in her voice, "but I didn't expect a brain transplant. He'll always be Eddie, he's trying really hard, and I love him more now than ever."

CHEMICAL COPING AND
PAIN MAGNIFICATION

Eddie's story highlights two critically important factors about emotions and their impact on chronic pain: chemical coping and pain magnification.

CHEMICAL COPING: Many of us, at a level below our conscious aware-ness, are medicating emotional pain that we perceive and experience as physical pain. Physical pain often begins the process—the sprained ankle, ruptured disk, migraine headache, strained tendon—but our emotions end up accelerating and intensifying the pain. As a result, when we take medication, we end up trying to numb both physical and emotional pain. When Eloise took Vicodin, for example, her joint pain eased up and she noticed that she was significantly less bothered by the kids running around the house, the dog barking, or her husband coming home late from work. When Stan realized he was running low on Per-cocet (prescribed for his rheumatoid arthritis) and might run out before his next refill, he was filled with anxiety—so he popped a few Xanax, to calm himself down. When Julianne took painkillers for chronic fatigue syndrome, they also helped numb her anguish over her husband's recent affair. And, clearly, as Eddie smothered both his chronic pain and his traumatic childhood memories in an opioid haze, his life became more tolerable, if just for a few hours.

PAIN MAGNIFICATION: Emotions are pain magnifiers. Our brain attaches special significance to emotionally charged events, which endure much longer in our memories and are recalled with greater accuracy than reg-ular, everyday experiences. Just for fun, think for a moment about why parrots swear. When their human owners curse, they are likely to put an unusual amount of emotional intensity into their words. Parrots are one of the few animals that can mimic human speech and because they feel, intuit, sense, or somehow latch onto the passion of our cursing, their brain (small and relatively uncomplicated as it is) flags the words as important and stores them in their long-term memory.

I once heard a story about Andrew Jackson, our country's tough, plain-spoken seventh president. According to legend, the president's foul-mouthed parrot continually interrupted his owner's stately funeral with nonstop cursing. The Reverend William Norment, who presided at the service, reported that the "wicked parrot . . . got excited and com-menced swearing so loud and long as to disturb the people . . . and let loose perfect gusts of 'cuss words.'" Mourners were "horrified and awed at the bird's lack of reverence."

This story, though a bit off-topic, illustrates the fact that strong emotions carry great weight (even in parrots), firing up the nervous system, triggering electrical and chemical signals that link to long-term memory. I wouldn't begin to profess expertise in the neurophysiology of parrots, but in humans I know that exciting or disturbing feelings agitate and activate the same areas of our brain that light up when we feel chronic physical pain. Painful experiences are *always*, inevitably emotional experiences.

When I first hurt my low back, I couldn't understand why the pain was so intense—all I had done was lean down to pick up a light suitcase! As I look back, I realize that I had been subconsciously wrestling with intense emotions. Hassling with my partner over finances and questioning whether the relationship should continue, grieving the death of a dear friend, and fretting over a conflict I was having with a co-worker had all taken their toll on my psyche. Thus, while the innocuous movement to lift my bag might have been the catalyst for the pain that followed, I'm pretty sure that it would have been unlikely to cause damage to my L4–L5 disks (discovered on an MRI a few months later) had I not been so anxious, distressed, and preoccupied for several weeks leading up to the event.

Just moments before I injured my back, I had an intense argument with a close friend. I was so angry I wanted to slug him and at the same time I felt guilty for losing my temper. My muscles were taut and tense and I was so upset with myself for getting into this predicament that I wonder now whether I subconsciously wanted to hurt myself as punishment for my bad judgment. At the time, I had none of these insights, but as I have looked back over the years at this truly life-changing event, it all makes perfect sense.

Now, almost ten years later, I reexperience back pain when I'm under stress at work or at home. Finances are always good for a nice back spasm! Or perhaps I'm fretting about a patient or a deadline, or sometimes, simply because it's Monday and I have a busy week ahead. When I feel tense and edgy, I often say some not-so-nice things to myself ("Slow down, what's wrong with you?," "It's only pain, for heaven's sake," "This is nothing compared to some of my patients," "Stop overreacting, you big baby").

Because I have been working with my emotions and their connection to my chronic pain for over a decade, I am soon able to take a different tack. I pause, take a few deep breaths, and recognize where my thoughts and feelings are taking me. Belatedly, I give my aching back a little relief with my orange massage ball and a good stretch, mentally preparing myself to drive to work in a calmer state of mind. Often I'll pull out the extra-large ice pack that's always ready in the freezer or call a trusted friend to discuss what's going on and search together for what is really bothering me. The biggest element in getting a handle on my pain is getting a handle on my emotional response, and I can do that by becoming aware of what I'm saying to myself and what emotions are coming up in the moment. The key is to notice these thoughts and emotions without judgment (more on this when we discuss mindfulness in Chapter 7).

THE PRIMARY EMOTIONS DRIVING CHRONIC PAIN

Let's briefly review the primary emotions driving chronic pain. As you read through these descriptions and stories, ask yourself which emotions seem to align most closely with your pain. Every emotion is linked with other emotions, so this process involves more than focusing on a clean-cut, clearly defined single emotion (e.g., Ken is frustrated, Debbie is anxious, Melinda is guilty, Stuart is ashamed).

Let's take Alex, for example, who is in a lot of pain after a fall from a ladder that shattered his ankle. He is furious with himself for getting on the ladder in the first place. His anger makes him anxious and when he is anxious, he is irritable and yells at his girlfriend. Then he feels guilty. Sadness and grief set in as he becomes acutely aware of how much he misses his children (grief) and suddenly shift to feelings of shame when he thinks about what a failure he is. And worst of all, he feels helpless to change his situation. His fear of having more pain rises and makes him feel even worse.

Anger causes anxiety and anxiety contributes to anger. Guilt and shame tend to meld together and it is often hard to tell which is which and what is what. Fear, anxiety, anger, guilt, grief, and helplessness are all cousins, and they like to congregate together much as cousins of the same age who may not particularly like one another might glom onto each other at a family reunion. And, like cousins, these emotions can grate on one another's nerves.

While all emotions circle around and cycle through our brain and body, for most of us one particular emotion will stand out as primary. Which of these powerful emotions might be driving your chronic pain?

Fear

"My heart was pounding so hard and I was so short of breath, that I actually thought I was having a heart attack," Gloria told me. "I honestly thought the man with the gun was going to shoot me."

When Gloria described the robbery that took place eight years earlier, shortly after her thirtieth birthday, the emotions she originally experienced played themselves out again as she told the story.

"I can't catch my breath and I'm so dizzy," she told me, her eyes wide and frightened. "I feel as if I'm right back in my apartment with that gun pointed at my head."

The robbers didn't shoot her but they threw her to the floor with such force that they fractured her ankle. "I've had three surgeries and the doctors eventually fused the bones," she said in a trembling voice. "I can't bend my ankle. And I'm in constant pain."

When she came into treatment, Gloria was taking six 10 mg Lortab for pain and four 2-mg Xanax tablets a day for anxiety and panic disorder. Withdrawal from the Lortab was tough enough, but stopping Xanax can be hellish and the protracted withdrawal can continue for weeks to months with anxiety, panic, racing heart, hot and cold sweats, tremors, and sleeplessness. Even after four weeks in treatment, Gloria was having difficulty adjusting to life without drugs and she was often flooded with fear, panic, and an ever-present feeling of being in grave, even mortal danger. She was hypervigilant, easily startled, had trouble sleeping, and often woke up in the night covered with sweat, her heart pounding.

Her greatest challenge was her tendency to catastrophize. "I'm so afraid that I'll never be able to walk without pain," she said with tears running down her cheeks and onto her lap. "Will the pain keep getting worse? Will I be disabled? Sometimes I think my ankle will just crumble underneath me and I'll spend the rest of my life on crutches or in a wheelchair. What's wrong with me? Am I a hypochondriac? Will I end up just like my mother, constantly moaning and groaning about her aching back?"

Over the course of six weeks in treatment, which included group therapy, individual counseling, gentle yoga, relaxation exercises, meditation, and deep breathing, Gloria's panic attacks eased and she was able to share her traumatic memories with her counselor and a few group members. Her pain became more manageable with each passing day as her body's natural painkillers kicked back in. And as she began to understand how her chronic pain was magnified by her fear and the painful memories related to the robbery, she spent many hours practicing various cognitive therapies designed to halt her catastrophic thinking before it cycled out of control.

"I have hope," she told me the day she left treatment. "And I'm not going to let fear rule my life anymore."

Of all our many varied, finely tuned emotions, fear has the most power to intensify our pain. I often refer to this quote by the well-known doctor and researcher Gordon Waddell: "Fear of pain and what we do about it may be more disabling than the pain itself." When we are afraid, our muscles tense and contract, which in turn increases the pressure on tender, hypersensitive, or damaged nerves. Fear makes our heart beat faster (or skip beats), we breathe harder (or we might hold our breath), we sweat, our stomach cramps, bowels loosen, we can't concentrate, we feel dizzy and unstable or frozen in place, and on and on it goes.

Fear is a trap for those of us living with chronic pain. Fearing that any little movement might cause more pain, we stop moving. We stop exercising. We stay home because we fear falling down the steps or tripping on the sidewalk. Some of us, as I've mentioned before, even fear getting out of bed to go to the bathroom. Our attempts to protect ourselves from pain by cutting back on any movement that might increase our pain trap us in a fear-avoidance syndrome (also called the unmovement syndrome; see page 137), which can seriously diminish not only our ability to move, as our muscles become stiff and frozen, but also our quality of life.

Of course, some fear is appropriate and keeps us from hurting ourselves (like the fear of walking too close to the edge of a cliff or driving recklessly). It's the inappropriate or unnecessary fear we sometimes experience that can create misery, isolation, anxiety, and depression. The question is—will you allow fear to transform your pain into suffering, shutting you off from the activities and the people you love? Or, stated another way, will you allow fear to rob you of a productive, joyful life?

The word *allow* is important, for while we cannot always control what happens to us, we can learn how to shut the door on "bad" un-necessary fear or at least hold onto it less tightly, thereby reducing our suffering. For suffering is optional—and, more importantly, can be re-solved more easily and successfully than fused bones or scar tissue.

Anxiety

Forty to 50 percent of chronic pain patients have symptoms of one of several common anxiety disorders: generalized anxiety disorder (con-stant worry, panic, or sudden, repeated attacks of fear), social anxiety (overwhelming anxiety in social situations), obsessive-compulsive dis-order (repeated thoughts or rituals that interfere with daily life), and/or post-traumatic stress disorder (repeated feelings of danger after a stress-ful event).

Although anxiety is appropriate when alerting us to real or per-ceived danger, it's not critical for the normal occurrences of our daily lives. When you have chronic pain, you get the double whammy—anxiety tends to intensify your pain and gnaw away at your quality of life, while the pain triggers anxiety (a positive feedback loop that is anything but positive). The upshot is, if your anxiety is severe and re-current, you can do something about it! (Several techniques described in Part 2 are particularly effective for anxiety, including exercise, medi-tation, breathing techniques, yoga, and Chi Kung.)

Harvey was an anxious guy—no one would argue that point; neither would he. He told me he was born nervous—a cranky, colicky baby; a poor sleeper; verbal and precocious from a young age. Today he would be diagnosed as oppositional and ADHD, most likely. He remembered his mother saying, "Why can't you be calm like your sister?," which set up a competitive relationship that would last a lifetime. He often wondered what was wrong with him, feeling somehow defective and unbalanced. Fast-forward fifty years to Harvey, age sixty-four. He was still a worrier, wringing his hands, tensing his jaw, and shaking his head negatively at any and all the suggestions I offered to teach him to worry less, which would in turn help him to tolerate his chronic pain from diabetic neuropathy.

"Anxiety is a negative rehearsal," I said one day. "You tell your-self bad things are going to happen and you feel awful whether or not they do. You are actually contributing to, if not creating, your own misery."

"Rehearsal?" he asked, incensed. "This is my life and it stinks. My feet hurt all the time—the neuropathy is killing me. And I'd be better off dead."

Harvey had a narrative in his mind that provoked his anxiety, with a good dose of fear thrown into the mix. "Once my feet start to hurt, *nothing will help!* I worry all the time—about my kids, and my wife's health. She had a heart attack, you know."

We went through this ritual on a daily basis. "When did your wife have her heart attack?" I asked.

"Thirty years ago, but you're a doctor, right?" Harvey answered, beginning to work himself up. "You know it can happen again! I couldn't survive twenty minutes without her!"

He also worried about money, even though he admitted one day that he had enough money to survive another lifetime. "But what if the market crashes?"

Harvey was an expert at getting himself worked up with a few words, and the tape in his mind would start running with dozens of "what if" scenarios. These racing thoughts plagued poor Harvey, causing him to gnaw on his fingernails and repeat his concerns over and over. Death was a constant source of anxiety, and he spoke often in group about death being "just around the corner."

One day, three weeks into treatment, a fellow group member blurted out in a fit of annoyance: "Come on Harvey—you're too mean to die!"

Harvey twisted in his chair with a shocked look and then suddenly burst out laughing. The whole group started laughing with him. Harvey laughed so hard tears were running down his cheeks. That was the day he truly began to change.

Anger and Resentment

Feeling hostile? Aggressive? Edgy? Want to bite someone's head off? Perhaps your own? Researchers confirm what all of us in chronic pain know from our own experience—we're angry. Pissed off. Livid. Frustrated because we're not getting what we want. Fed up.

A recent study found that nearly 40 percent of chronic pain patients are angry—generally angry, aggressive, hostile, angry at themselves, the world, all of the above. Here comes that double whammy once again—patients who are angry have significantly higher levels of anxiety and pain. And there's another twist to this anger story—those of us who inhibit or who are unable to honestly and openly express our negative, rage-filled emotions experience greater pain.

Lily had no problem whatsoever venting her anger; she was a very difficult, ornery, generally unlikeable person to be around.

"I'm too old for this crap," Lily, 62, said, her brown eyes blazing.

We'd been talking about the problems she was having with her roommate and other patients at the center, and I told her she simply had to get her anger under control or we would have to ask her to leave. She was holding grudges, refusing to talk in group, spreading rumors, and complaining about everything—including me.

"You're angry with me," I said, stating the obvious. Her response surprised me.

"I'm mad at you and everyone else because I want to get back to the way I was before that damn accident," she said in a moment of absolute honesty. "If you can't help me return to my old life, the hell with you all."

When I asked her to write in her journal about her anger and how her resentments might be increasing her pain ("Is there a reason you might be holding onto your pain?" I asked), she stormed out of my office, muttering just loud enough for me to hear, "Go f— yourself." I heard her shouting in the hallway, "That doctor is crazy and I want to go home . . . now!" As she passed by open doors in the hallway, she slammed them shut and the jarring sound reverberated through the entire treatment center.

Lily's father had sexually molested her from the time she was three until age nine, when she summoned up the courage to tell her grandmother. After that, she lived with her maternal grandparents until she graduated from high school and although they doted on her, they never spoke to her again about the abuse, and told her to never discuss it again—with anyone. In her journal, Lily confessed that she felt as if she had a "deep dark scar on my soul." A hard worker and brilliant student, Lily attended an Ivy League college and a prestigious law school. She married, had two children, and managed a successful career. After she was sworn to secrecy by her grandmother, she had never told another living soul what her father had done to her—until she came to treatment.

When she slipped on an icy sidewalk and shattered two vertebrae in her neck, her doctor prescribed opioids at higher and higher doses for pain. Her psychiatrist prescribed Klonipen for anxiety, along with several antidepressants. "Anything to shut me up," she told me. "My back surgeon couldn't wait to get me out of the office—he was always good for a prescription of one hundred and twenty Percocets. And the quack at the pain clinic prescribed the morphine."

Lily came into treatment after a suicide attempt. She immediately began picking fights with other patients and staff members. Most of the patients avoided her and she often ate alone in a corner of the cafeteria. "Most people don't like me," she admitted. "I don't blame them—I know I scare them off. It's easier that way—I can reject them before they reject me. That's been my way for a long time. It works." But was it really working?

Lily often astonished me with her honesty and insight. She realized that she had pushed people away her whole life, and she was open to the idea of being less aggressive, softening up a bit, even apologizing to people at the center whom she had offended. "I do have a gentle side," she admitted at one point. "Deep down, I'm a real sweetheart. It's just that when I'm not angry, I feel vulnerable and I worry so much about getting hurt that I shut those feelings down."

Lily, like Eddie, was a good example of the clinical maxim "Hurt people hurt people." Over time she was able to see how anger affected both her pain level and her emotional and psychological health. With the drugs out of her system, she discovered a new willingness to participate in group and individual therapy and she devoted hours every day to journal and free writing. Toward the end of treatment, she participated in a forgiveness group, which had a profound effect on her.

"Resentments are like alley cats—they only stay around if you feed them," she said with a twinkle in her eye. "Did you know that the word *resentment* comes from the French word *resentir*, which means 'to feel again'?" she asked me another day. "So, my resentments made me feel the pain over and over again, and I let it consume me."

I shared with Lily one of my favorite Buddha quotes. "Holding on to anger is like grasping a hot coal with the intent of throwing it at someone else; you are the one who gets burned."

Guilt

Everybody I have ever met who has chronic pain feels as if he or she did something to deserve it.

Mark was just twenty-six years old and working as a firefighter when he arrived at the scene of a car accident. One of the cars crashed through a bridge railing and ended up in the river below. Mark dove into the water and saved the driver, but her sixteen-month-old baby drowned.

A few months later, Mark injured his neck in an accident when he fell from a ladder during a training exercise. He immediately developed excruciating pain that, it turned out, was from a ruptured disk. After two unsuccessful surgeries, his surgeon and primary care physician prescribed long-acting morphine with immediate-release morphine for breakthrough pain, eventually taking a total daily dose of 700 mg of morphine.

Mark toughed it out for twenty years but the pain and disability eventually took their toll. No longer able to work as a firefighter, he was relegated to teaching new recruits, but he had trouble sustaining that job as well because he was on such high doses of morphine. He was also seriously depressed. When he "accidentally" overdosed on his medications, his wife and two daughters worried that he had intentionally ingested extra pills. They arranged for an intervention and he agreed to go to treatment but only, he told me, "for them."

After a rough, ten-day detox, Mark was free of opioid medications for the first time in twenty years. But even though he felt more alert and his pain levels were significantly reduced, he was unusually irritable and depressed.

"I keep dreaming about a car accident that happened over twenty years ago," he told me. "I have nightmares where I see a baby drowning underwater and I can't reach her."

Over time, as he repeated the story and experienced the emotions that had been repressed and sublimated by the opioids, he was able to accept the fact that there was nothing he could have done that would have saved the baby. He eventually came to the understanding that part of his drive to take the drugs was to smother his guilt and his shame for being inadequate.

"I feel guilty because I couldn't save the baby," he told me in a moment of great insight. "But I feel ashamed because I wasn't strong enough, I didn't react quickly enough—I wasn't good enough to save that child's life. I always believed that I was responsible, I was to blame for that death." Of course, that simply wasn't true and he finally was able to see the truth.

When Mark was able to think clearly and talk openly about his emotions, now that he was off the painkilling, mind-numbing drugs, he was able to forgive himself. "I realize that I did the best I could," he told me. "I would have given my life for that child. But there was nothing I could do—there was nothing anyone could have done—to save her."

With that emerging sense of self-forgiveness, Mark's pain virtually disappeared. When he left treatment, he told me his pain level was zero.

Guilt is such a driving emotional force in chronic pain that two more stories may help highlight its significance in treatment and recovery. Guy was driving a car and was involved in a head-on collision; he woke up from a coma three weeks later to learn that his wife had been killed in the accident. He had lost control of the car because he looked away momentarily and that was the last thing he remembered. He was sixty-eight years old and still practicing medicine at the time. A year after the accident, he developed severe, unrelenting headaches. His pain was so severe that he was forced to quit work. His physician prescribed fentanyl patches, increasing the dose to 75 mcg every two days (a very high dose). His pain subsided but so did his ability to function, and his son, an only child, finally intervened.

"I cannot allow you to be with your grandson in the state you are in," his son told him. Faced with the reality of losing the only family he had left, Guy entered treatment.

Even after two weeks in treatment, Guy rated his headache pain as a steady 7 or 8 out of 10. He became frustrated and discouraged as he saw everybody around him getting better while he felt he wasn't improving at all. In a counseling session, he confided that he felt responsible for his wife's death but his guilt was compounded by the fact that he'd been having an affair with his wife's best friend for several years before the accident. The next day he rated his pain as a 6; a week later, it was a 4. Encouraged by his counselor, Guy wrote a letter to his dead wife, asking her to forgive him, and from that point on he was ready to move on with his life.

Helen was driving drunk and broke her left ankle in four places. She soon became dependent on methadone prescribed for pain, and

Valium, prescribed for anxiety and panic attacks. She felt responsible for her own injury and the injuries of the passengers in her car. When asked about letting go of her pain, she said she felt she didn't deserve to be free of pain. "The pain is my just reward for being so foolish and irresponsible," she confessed. Only after many hours of therapy did she begin to pry herself loose from the grip of guilt about what she had done. Little by little, she was able to see that forgiving herself would free her to return to a productive life and begin the work of making amends to the people she had hurt.

When I think about Mark, Guy, and Helen, I realize that they have been able to assimilate and incorporate into their lives the simple truth of this Buddhist saying: "Pain is not a punishment. Joy is not a reward. They are simply occurrences."

Grief

Living with chronic pain means living with loss. You grieve the loss of your "old self," the person you thought you were or would become. You come face to face with your limitations and your inability to turn the clock back, to regain that old self whom you look back on now with profound sadness. Where did you go? How did this happen? Why can't you change it, alter it, make it go away?

These questions haunt virtually every person who lives with chronic pain. Once again, as with guilt, anxiety, anger, fear, and so many intense emotions, the questions we ask ourselves point to an existential angst—our inability to control or predict what has happened to us. We lose hope in the future as our losses pile up—loss of health, work, relationships with friends and family members, vitality, energy and, potentially, loss of many years of quality in our life. With every doctor visit, every new diagnosis, every additional pill, every argument with a family member, every friend who abandons us, we grieve. Our grief is palpable—it thickens the air of the world we live in—and yet we do everything we can to stuff it inside, hide it away, and smother the life out of it. For to recognize or acknowledge that we are grieving would mean having to face the depth and breadth of our loss.

It is helpful for people with chronic pain to consider Elisabeth Kübler-Ross's five stages of grief in the process of death and dying—denial, anger, bargaining, depression, and acceptance—and how relevant these stages are to their own experience. Diana, 70, has fibromyalgia and has been living with chronic pain for fifteen years (we first met Diana in Chapter 1). She explains how cycling through the stages of grief lead her to question the very meaning of life. What meaning is there in the pain? What's the point, what's the purpose?

▪ If chronic, long-term pain patients face constantly changing body circumstances, and therefore deal with grief nearly all the time, how does one do that and still have a life? Living long years in chronic pain and losing losing losing is really just doing the steps of grieving over and over again. There is no end to grief work when you live in this kind of life. Because just when you think, "Well thank God that's done, I won't have to deal with that again," you are in sweet acceptance. But then when another giant loss or embarrassment comes along, you have to start all over again with denial, anger, bargaining, and depression.

With death there is a beginning, a middle, and an end to the stages. But not with chronic pain. You are constantly in one stage or another because the body gets sicker or the pain gets worse or a friend leaves who just can't take it anymore. There is no way out of the stages of grieving in this chronic pain life. *That* is the source of deep hopelessness. Learning how to live with hopelessness is a challenge. I will always be in one grief stage or another!

How does one do the necessary grief work yet stay in a positive mind-set? Because if chronic, long-term pain patients face constantly changing body circumstances and therefore need to do grief work nearly all the time—how does one do that and still have a life?

I was sitting in my chair, not really thinking, just reading and playing on my iPad, when I realized tears were quietly falling from my eyes— that horrible weeping from one's soul. I stopped and thought back to the morning trying to figure out what had caused the weeping—it didn't take long to realize what caused me such grief. That morning, my sweet dog needed to go outside for a walk, and I could not walk her past our backyard. My hips and legs were hurting badly. I stood in the front yard and thought, "I can't even take my dog for a short walk."

At that point, I see and hear another door in my life slam shut. But I am glad I can recognize grief so fast because I am familiar with the signs. I can be sad and grieve and I can begin to work through the stages of grief again, from denial to anger to bargaining to depression and, finally, to acceptance. To be chronically ill for a long, long time is basically perpetual grieving. I know it is never over. I weep. And I move on.

▓ ▓ ▓

Helplessness

Helplessness is usually viewed by medical professionals as a symptom of depression. But I have come to believe that helplessness is a primary emotion in chronic pain patients and contributes mightily to depression, anxiety, fear, anger, loneliness, guilt, shame, and, of course, hopelessness. Helplessness may, in fact, be predictive of depression.

When we are in chronic pain, we feel helpless. We believe there is little or nothing we can do to change the difficult situation. Try as we might to control our life, pain has the final word. Pain *always* has the final word, or so it seems, and over time we may begin to see ourselves as victims, whiners, complainers, losers, lost causes. Our helplessness in the face of unrelenting chronic pain gnaws away at our very sense of self and any faith we might have in our ability to alter our situation. Over time, we become so discouraged about having no way to escape that we feel downtrodden, depressed, hopeless, and despairing.

In a series of classic but brutal experiments conducted more than forty years ago (such experiments could not be conducted today because of strong ethical standards for animal and human research), psychologist Martin Seligman and his colleagues subjected German shepherds to painful electric shocks. In the first experiments, the dogs were placed in a restraining harness and received the shocks day and night. At first, the dogs tried mightily to escape, straining against their harness, howling, growling, urinating. But as the shocks continued no matter what they did or how hard they struggled, the dogs "learned" to stop resisting. With no way to escape, they simply resigned themselves to the pain. This was their life. This was the way it would always be.

The image of a helpless dog subjected to constant electric shocks, whimpering in a corner, completely submissive and accepting of its fate is haunting and deeply disturbing. In later experiments the same German shepherds did have a way to escape the pain—all they had to do was jump over a low barrier to the other side of the box, where they would be insulated from the shocks. Instead, they curled up in a corner of their cage, whimpering with each electric jolt. They had "learned" to stop fighting. They had "learned" to accept their fate of constant, unrelieved pain.

Chronic pain delivers random, electric jolts that all too often lead to a sense of helplessness in humans. We struggle and fight back, trying everything within our command to stop the pain, but over time it wears us down. Perhaps you have had an experience like the German shepherd cowering in the corner of the cage, whimpering, accepting the pain because you see no way to escape from it. Once again, this is a haunting image, and I have seen the "picture" too often in my interactions with patients who have simply given up any hope of a better life.

Are you "harnessed" or tethered to your pain? Have you learned that no matter what you do, the pain cannot be escaped? After months and years of struggling against the pain, have you resigned yourself to a life of constant, unrelenting chronic pain? What are the consequences of such resignation? Perhaps you can relate to Marie's story.

My husband was driving too fast on the icy roads. We were headed up the mountain to ski when he took a corner, skidded, and rolled the car off the side of the road. I spent two weeks in the hospital after surgery to repair my spinal injuries, but over the next few years the pain just got worse.

I took painkillers, muscle relaxants, antidepressants, and anti-anxiety drugs, all prescribed by my doctor. I had a second surgery and I'll never forget what the surgeon said six months later when I told him the pain was as bad as ever. "The surgery was successful, everything looks great, there's nothing more we can do for you."

That's when I found myself sinking into a dark and awful place. I saw myself as a helpless, worthless, pathetic shell of a human being. I deeply resented my husband for causing the accident that left me a weak, whimpering invalid. I quit my job, cut myself off from all my friends, and spent most of my days in bed wanting to die because life hurt too much. It wasn't just physical pain—it felt like something was gnawing away at my heart and soul.

For me, those feelings of helplessness translate into existential questions about my reason for being. What is my purpose here? When I am in pain and can't get away from it, the fear and anxiety come rushing in and I wonder what is the point of being here, on this earth? I question who I am and I also wonder who would want to be around this whiny invalid, this weak mess of a human being. The negative voices are so loud. The more I try to quiet myself, the more I hear these loud voices telling me, "You are not enough," and I want to run as fast as I can so I can stay busy, so I can ignore these voices. But at the same time my aching physical body is saying, "You have to rest."

I need a new story to tell myself. My old story is not working, I know that but I don't know how to stop it, I don't know how to stop the anger at myself for not being able to heal my body even after taking classes, participating in workshops, massages, acupuncture, reading self-help books, trying to find the next fix-it book, searching, searching. I feel that I have to go within for these answers—I have to go into my emotions and ask what triggers me, I have to look at what patterns run my life—perfectionism, victimhood, being a goody-goody and a pleaser, always feeling guilty when I have the pain.

What did I do to deserve this? I isolate because I don't have the energy to be around anyone, it takes too much energy to engage with others. I just want to suffer alone. I can't hide the pain from others and who wants to be around me like this? I crawl home to my safe place, my nest, and I lay there and lick my wounds praying that when I wake up this will be gone.

There is so much inside of me that I don't know where to begin . . .

▪ ▪ ▪

SUFFERING IS OPTIONAL

There are two kinds of suffering: the suffering that leads to
more suffering and the suffering that leads to the end of suffering.
If you are not willing to face the second kind of suffering,
you will surely continue to experience the first.

—AJAHN CHAH, *A STILL FOREST POOL*

Several years ago I attended a retreat at Esalen in Northern California, led by Jon Kabat-Zinn and his son Ben Zinn. One day during a break, I screwed up my courage and went up to the stage. Jon was very approachable, but still I felt a bit like a groupie when I introduced myself and sat down next to him. I told him how important his work had been in developing the pain program at LVRC and we talked about the challenges of helping people who live with chronic pain, a topic close to both our hearts.

"You know, Mel, the thing that is most important when I work with people is that they know *there is more right with them than wrong with them*. So, I tell them this, regularly."

I knew these words by heart—I'd memorized them from Jon's book *Full Catastrophe Living*—but to hear them spoken out loud by this gentle, soulful man had a great impact on me.

Suffering results from the state of mind where you believe that there is more wrong with you than right with you. For many people living with chronic pain, suffering comes from the belief that there is *nothing* right with you. Those beliefs gradually build seemingly insurmountable barriers that separate and isolate you from others and from yourself. For if so much is wrong with you, if nothing is right with you, then you do not deserve love, compassion, attention, and comforting words. You are set apart, undeserving, unworthy. Indeed, "I am not worthy of love" is the conscious or subconscious thought that lives and breathes at the very heart of suffering.

Not so very long ago, I was talking with patients in a group session at the treatment center. I asked a question I often ask: "Why is it that we know the things that are good for us, but we don't do them?" Most often the answer is, "Oh, I'm just lazy," "I can't get motivated," or "I get so busy that I forget." But Donald, a philosophy professor from Oregon, diagnosed with fibromyalgia years earlier, offered something different.

"I don't deserve to be comfortable," he said. "I don't deserve to take this time for myself, to meditate, walk, reflect, write, exercise, all the things you are asking us to do. I'm not worthy of my own time because I have too many other people I need to think about and take care of." Donald's statement took the group by surprise because he was such a cerebral guy, always deep in thought, contributing to the group only when he felt the need to espouse some philosophical or theoretical belief.

I wanted to respond by saying, "And how's that going for you?," but I restrained myself. That was the imperfect side of me rising up in impatience, wanting to challenge Donald to look at himself and gain some insight into what was really going on inside him. Donald would do that in his own time, in his own way. It was necessary work, for those words and that mind-set, "I don't deserve to be comfortable . . . or happy . . . or content . . . or take time for myself . . . " are not the basis for living well—and, in fact, often form the foundation for our persistent misery. Some of the feedback he heard from the group was along those lines, whereas a number of his fellow patients expressed gratitude for his honesty and identified similar thoughts and feelings.

In treatment Donald would learn the strategies and techniques that would help him realize that we all deserve to be comfortable, happy, and content, and to do that we need to take time for ourselves. I sincerely hoped that he would continue to use what he had learned to let go of the intensity of his discomfort and find a way to live and thrive with his chronic pain. It was encouraging that he was willing to be so open, honest, and vulnerable—a good first step to getting better.

Another common excuse for not exercising, meditating, eating well, stretching, reading, resting, writing, reflecting—all the "good" things we can do to fill ourselves up when we are empty and drained—is "It's too hard," or "I just don't have the energy." As you read this book, consider this question: If you know what's good for you—good in the sense of nurturing, strengthening, enlivening you—what holds *you* back from taking care of yourself on a regular basis? Why is it so hard to do the things that strengthen and sustain you? Exercising when you have chronic pain certainly can be uncomfortable. But if you have been taught to take care of your body, mind, and spirit so as not to fall victim to anger and anxiety, to combat negative thoughts and attitudes so as not to become overwhelmed by hopelessness and helplessness, to engage with the world rather than retreat into a lonely, isolated place where you can lick your wounds, then why do you leave those lessons behind and fall back into harmful behaviors?

So again, I ask myself, and I ask you to ask yourself: Why do we human beings shy away from doing things that are good for us? The answer to that fascinating question comes down to one simple fact—we are human. In other words, we are not perfect. All we can do is keep trying.

Let me tell you a story about a young man who came into treatment a few years ago with severe, unrelenting pain related to a terrifying, life-threatening condition—a brain tumor known as **astrocytoma**.

JASON'S STORY

■ "I don't want to be alive," Jason said.

I waited for him to continue but he simply glared at me. I think he expected me to comfort or reassure him that he should want to live, but I sensed that he needed to put those words out there and not be contradicted. So, we sat together as he choked up—his suffering was strong and thick and I felt my own throat closing and my eyes tearing. I knew that I could not convince him of his own self-worth nor make life meaningful for him. That conviction had to come from inside him, just as his belief that he was unworthy and undeserving came from inside him. He believed, right to the core of his being, that he did not deserve this second chance at life.

"Why did I survive surgery for this brain tumor when most people die?"

Jason had done his homework. "Did you know that sixty percent of people with similar tumors would be dead?" he asked me. "And of those who live through it, two out of three have permanent neurological problems or disabilities? I'm only thirty-two years old; most people with this condition are much older. Why did this happen to me?" I didn't articulate out loud the thought that popped into my head: *Why not you?*

"The tumor or the headaches?" I asked. Jason suffered from headaches that were so fiercely debilitating that he spent much of the day in a darkened room. After detoxing him from large doses of OxyContin (400 mg per day) and Percocet (260 mg per day), Jason was relieved to be off the opioids ("They made me a vegetable"), but his headaches were still 9 out of 10 on the pain scale. I was pretty sure that he was holding on to his pain—but why? What purpose did it serve for him?

"I'm so tired of the headaches, the total body pain, having a tumor—take your pick," Jason said with undisguised anger. "I'm sick of talking about my feelings and listening to all of these complainers in group all day long. They have such sad stories, I just can't stand it. I listen to their stories and after group I just feel worse. I want to throw up. All these stories, all this pain make my head hurt worse. Don't you understand? I don't want to do this. I can't do this!"

Jason pointed at his chest, his face contorted, eyes narrowed, mouth twisted and then began to pound on the desk with his fist. He was pounding so hard, I winced in mirrored pain. "I can't stand this anymore. I hate myself. I need to get the hell out of here. I have to get back on OxyContin and Percocet, even if the drugs made me a vegetable, they were the only thing that worked to kill the pain. I don't understand why I can't have the pills, I just took them for the pain, that's all, I never snorted them or injected them, I did just what my doctor told me to do."

I felt the need to respond as he had worked himself into a highly agitated state. "But you were shooting heroin for the last few months, Jason," I said calmly.

"I only did heroin because the doctor reduced my dose of Oxys and Percs and wouldn't give me anything to sleep, so when the pain got worse, I went to the street. What would you have done, Doc?"

I didn't respond to his question, knowing he didn't really want an answer from me. After a few moments he put his head in his hands and massaged his temples. When he looked up, his eyes were red, either from stuffing back the tears or from the intensity of his physical pain.

Jason left two days later, after just six days in treatment. His suffering was related to his anger and sense of victimization—*Why me?*— and behind that anger, feeding and enlarging it, was the fear that he would not be able to manage his life successfully without painkillers. He suffered because he wanted things to be different. He wanted to use drugs and not be addicted to them. He wanted to be "normal" and not have to deal with pain that never went away. He suffered because he believed he would be in pain every minute of every day of his life, that he would need opioids forever, that the world was meaningless, life sucked, and worst of all, that nothing would ever change. He felt victimized by his body, his parents, and the treatment center. And for all of that, he felt deep, searing shame believing that he was deficient, inadequate, worthless.

There was no meaning to anything, Jason believed, no sense at all to life and therefore no reason to try to move through suffering and transcend it. Because where would he go, then, what place would offer him comfort, who could ever truly care about him or love him when the real problem was that he was a "piece of crap." The way Jason figured it, he'd still be a "piece of crap" even if he was off drugs and out of pain. At that point in time, and perhaps for many months or years to come, he would believe he wasn't worth the time and the effort it would take to change.

■ ■ ■

WINNING BY LOSING

Jason held onto his pain because it shielded him from the reality that drugs were not the solution. His pain was so bad that he convinced himself he *had* to take drugs. Otherwise, he believed, he was suffering just for the sake of suffering. Was it fair to try to wean him off the drugs when they were the only thing that stood between him and his pain? Yes, because the drugs had stopped working—he had to use more and more to alleviate his pain and the numbness lasted only a short time. The drugs had imprisoned him in his pain and were gnawing away at the quality of his life. And yet they also offered him an hour or two of blessed relief, and he couldn't bear to let go of that brief respite from the physical, mental, and spiritual pain. So, that's where he focused, on the few minutes or hours when he was numb and temporarily liberated from pain.

Jason also embraced his pain because it gave him an identity—"chronic pain victim." He believed he deserved to suffer—he had a brain tumor, he almost died, and in his opinion, he *should* have died. Who could ask for a better reason to suffer and to continue suffering?

But perhaps most important of all, Jason held fast to his pain and his drugs because without them, he was vulnerable, naked, exposed. The pain gave him an excuse to hide away, to continue to believe that life had no meaning, to turn his face to the wall and his back to people who cared about him. Part of his misery was his existential belief that he didn't deserve a pain-free life—suffering was his deserved fate. Paradoxically his isolation was soothing to him—he didn't have to think about anything but himself and his own suffering. He didn't have to face (at least not squarely) his emotions, his fear, his terror. Believing that he lived in a world without meaning allowed him to stay in that world and avoid the more difficult and challenging journey—finding significance and a sense of self in a life edged by pain, rather than in the people who loved him, cared for him, and would do anything within their power to help him.

SECONDARY GAIN

Jason won by losing. This is called secondary gain—the unconscious benefits we receive from our suffering. Those of us living with chronic pain do not purposefully look to gain anything from our pain, but we are often rewarded in some way for our suffering.

"Rewarded" for pain and suffering? I know—this is a really tough concept to accept. It is critically important to understand that we do not "ask for" or "cause" our pain. With or without our conscious knowledge, however, we experience certain benefits because we are having pain and we respond, often without awareness, to the positive energy (compassion, caring, and concern). Often we are relieved of responsibilities and spared certain stressors ("No, dear, I'll go shopping, you stay and rest," or "You're exhausted, let me prepare dinner and bring it to you in bed"). In a very real sense, we become conditioned to the positives that accompany our pain and maybe even to the experience of subconsciously wanting to hold onto the pain we have—even though, truly, we would give anything to be rid of pain.

I know from my work with hundreds of patients that when you are able to see and understand the role of secondary gain in creating and extending your suffering, your awareness will help you "un-hook" yourself from a sense of victimhood. I also know this from my own experience of chronic pain. When I injured my back in 2003, the pain was excruciating—but all I did was lean down to pick up a carry-on bag! I was actually relieved when the MRI showed a bulging disk because now I had an excuse to be in so much pain. And as much as I hate to admit it, in some odd way, the pain I was experiencing and the consequences of having that pain had some surprising advantages. Although I wasn't consciously rewarding myself for having pain, I had a really legitimate reason to take it easy and avoid exercise. I had a great excuse to sit around and watch TV, and, of course I had to eat while I was watching TV, which gave me an acceptable justification for gaining weight. After all, I was in pain.

In most of my conversations with friends and family, the opening line was, "How's your back?" A well-timed groan or moan, more often than not, elicited the sought-after sympathetic "poor Melly . . ."

Now at the time, if you told me that any of this served me, I would have slugged you. After all, I was hurting, frustrated, angry, and miserable most of the time. I felt helpless, powerless, and hopeless. How could anyone suggest I was benefiting from my pain? Thankfully, not a soul dared to make such a suggestion because, without question, that would have given me a great excuse to bite someone's head off. And I needed an excuse—any excuse—to yell and scream; I was looking for a reason to snap.

It took me a long time to realize that as long as I remained angry and frustrated, my muscles stayed tight. The longer I stayed inactive, the less attractive activity seemed (I was stuck in the *unmovement syndrome*, which you will learn more about later). The more I ate, the more weight I gained, and the more weight I gained, the worse I felt about myself. My lack of self-worth gave me a good excuse—the best of excuses!—to wallow around in my suffering (and have another bowl of ice cream).

Today, more than a decade later, my pain is still there, but it is bearable. What changed? I got tired of the pain, of complaining, and of being miserable. I realized that my identity was wrapped around my back pain, and I had become locked in the vicious cycle of a futile search for freedom from chronic pain, which only caused me more suffering. When I resisted the pain—with anger, frustration, bitterness, resentment—the agony worsened. I began to understand that my heated emotions actually fueled my pain. Over time, I learned to stop fighting and judging the pain (and judging myself for having the pain). And, lo and behold, the pain lessened for hours and sometimes days at a time. When I stopped fighting the pain, when I "let go" and called a cease-fire to the attempt to change what cannot be changed—when I surrendered—the pain lessened. It didn't go away, but I didn't fret so much about it.

I'm often comforted by Kahlil Gibran's quote, "Out of suffering have emerged the strongest souls; the most massive characters are seared with scars." We've all got our scars, that's for sure. And the truth is that it is hard to let go of our suffering. We get "hooked" by physical pain and by the emotions that accompany the painful stimulus. Anything that touches the tender places—the aching, raw spots—can grab us and capture our wholehearted attention. We tense up at the sensation—that tightening and clenching is involuntary, not under our conscious control—and then we feel the urge to move away, to flee from the pain, to seek relief from the discomfort. Of course, this urge to experience relief is more than just "seeking"—it is a drive, a powerful force within us that craves release from the pain and yearns for freedom from the anguish, anxiety, and agitation that seem to never leave us alone.

Maybe we turn to food. Or work. Or shopping. Or sex. Or alcohol, or other drugs. We are looking for anything that will restore a sense of well-being or, more accurately, offer a short-term reprieve and some consolation for our misery. But no matter how much we bury ourselves in food, work, material possessions, sex, or drugs, when we come up for air the pain is still there. These measures are more of the same—compulsive behaviors to escape from the inescapable truth: it hurts.

Suffering can be hard to wrap your head around in this—or, in truth, in any—context, for suffering resides in the heart and soul, in that place deep inside where we wonder where we fit and belong. Suffering calls into question our very purpose in life, our reason for "being." Thus, one of the most effective ways to deal with suffering is to confront it head on, asking what it wants from you and what purpose it serves for you. Here are two exercises to help you better understand your suffering and, over time, let go of its hold over you.

Secondary Gain

Think honestly and openly about the points below. Can you identify any hidden "benefits" you might receive from your pain and suffering?

- **Physical:** I can rest, relax, take it easy. I don't have to exercise and I always hated it anyway. I don't have to help around the house (mowing the lawn, taking out the garbage, doing the taxes, cooking, cleaning, grocery shopping . . .)
- **Social:** If I'm late to an event or have to cancel at the last moment, everyone will understand. My family and friends will make excuses for me. (I never enjoyed social events anyway.)
- **Emotional:** I'm angry, irritable, and moody because I'm in so much pain. I can get away with my emotional outbursts. People pay attention to me ("How are you feeling?" "Is there anything I can do for you?"). I have a reasonable excuse to use painkilling drugs.
- **Relational:** My family and friends pay more attention to me when my pain is intense or out of control, or they leave me alone when I need to rest. My children will understand why I need to stay home and sleep or watch TV rather than go to their athletic games when my arthritis is acting up. I can't cook meals anymore (and I've always hated cooking).
- **Professional:** I have a right to call in sick when I'm in a lot of pain—after all, there's no way I can work when my pain flares up. I have an excuse to miss work all together ("Early retirement!" "Workers comp or disability!" "Use up all those sick day benefits!").
- **Financial:** I receive disability, and although I make less money than I did when I worked, why should I work when I get paid for not working? How can I risk going back to work and giving up these payments? What if I go back to work and can't hack it? (I'll stick with disability, thanks.)
- **Sexual:** I'm just too exhausted to have sex; it hurts too much to be touched; and my partner understands. Since I've been on the meds, I've lost interest and have a good excuse not to participate.

Ask Yourself . . .

Questions that may help relieve your suffering:

- What is suffering trying to communicate to me? Fill in the blank in this sentence. I suffer because _____ [I'm lonely, nobody understands, there's no hope . . .].
- Might suffering be a means to an end, pointing not to the problem but to the solution? I am lonely—is there something I can do to ease my loneliness? Nobody understands—is it possible that someone does understand but doesn't know how to help? Would it help to talk to other people with chronic pain or join a group, such as Pain in Recovery Support Group (PIRSG)? If there is indeed no hope for an end to chronic pain, what then? How do I come to terms with my life as it is?
- Are there things that I do or attitudes that I have that enlarge and expand my suffering? For example, do I fight the pain, wishing it away, denying its existence? Do I cling to the past, wishing that things could be the way they used to be and feeling sad and dejected because I'm not the way I used to be? Am I afraid of the future and have I convinced myself that the pain will only get worse?
- Of the emotions most commonly associated with chronic pain—fear, anxiety, anger/resentment, guilt, grief, and helplessness—which emotion is most connected with my pain? Is this emotion helpful or hurtful? Is there anything I can do to lessen its negative impact on my life?
- How am I resisting my pain? How does resisting the pain make it worse and increase my suffering? What can I do to decrease my resistance?
- Which memories tend to trigger my suffering? What can I do to "unhook" myself from those memories, freeing myself from the past so that I can live more fully in the present?
- What would it be like to feel my pain without judging it?
- What would it be like to look straight into the heart of my pain rather than averting my eyes or trying to shield myself from pain and my fears about the future?

FOUR

AM I ADDICTED?

Understanding the Difference Between Dependence and Addiction

I had a doctor who I greatly respect mention to me that,
you know, we thought the big problem with these
drugs was addiction. What we didn't realize is that
people who take them would opt out of life.

—BARRY MEIER

Chances are pretty good that if you are in chronic pain, you are taking, have taken, or have been offered opioid drugs. (For a list of these drugs, see www.thepainantidote.com.) Like their chemical cousin heroin, prescription opioids have the potential to be fiercely addicting. If you take opioids steadily for more than one month, you are likely to become dependent upon them.

But will you become addicted to them? This brings us to questions that most people living with chronic pain would rather avoid, given the fact that these potent painkillers seem to offer the only hope for truly effective pain relief:

- What, exactly, is addiction?
- How do I know if I'm addicted to the drugs I take for pain relief?
- What is the difference between addiction and dependence?
- What is "complex dependence"?

ADDICTION

Let's look, first, at how we define *addiction*. I recently served on a committee of the American Society of Addiction Medicine (ASAM) that developed a comprehensive definition to thoroughly explain the fact that addiction is a true medical disease—a disease of the brain. The definition doesn't just include drug addiction but also encompasses "behavioral" or "process" addictions (food, sex, shopping, gambling, Internet) and the brain pathology underlying these behaviors. Previous definitions of addiction defined behaviors that are symptomatic of the disease but didn't explain what goes wrong inside the brain and body to give rise to those behaviors. The ASAM definition is a great improvement over these earlier versions because it explores the neurobiology of addiction and the bio-psycho-socio-spiritual nature of the disease, which I believe is crucial to understanding recovery.

Most people don't have the energy or desire to wade through the long version (no wonder, it's 2,879 words); here is an abbreviated version:

> Addiction is a primary, chronic disease of brain reward, motivation, memory and related circuitry. Dysfunction in these circuits leads to characteristic biological, psychological, social and spiritual manifestations. This is reflected in an individual pathologically pursuing reward and/or relief by substance use and other behaviors.
>
> Addiction is characterized by inability to consistently abstain, impairment in behavioral control, craving, diminished recognition of significant problems with one's behaviors and interpersonal relationships, and a dysfunctional emotional response. Like other chronic diseases, addiction often involves cycles of relapse and remission. Without treatment or engagement in recovery activities, addiction is progressive and can result in disability or premature death.

If that's a mouthful, I've stripped the whole thing down to what I consider its most fundamental parts: *Addiction is the pathological pursuit of relief and/or reward.*

Even this supershort version can be confounding, however, so let me tease it apart into its various components.

PATHOLOGICAL: This is a tough concept for many people to understand and it is particularly difficult for those of us in chronic pain—for what may appear "pathological" to some may also seem perfectly legitimate to people seeking relief from unrelenting physical discomfort. The particular drug you use and your reasons for using it may also skew the picture. For example, while it may seem unreasonable or extreme to pop Xanax regularly during the day to deal with anxiety or stress, taking high doses of Vicodin or Percocet might be viewed as a legitimate strategy to reduce the everyday agony of chronic pain.

So, what do we mean by "pathological"? Pathology indicates a disease state and pathological refers to behavior that is caused by or related to a mental or physical disease. Victims of leprosy can run for miles on a broken ankle because the disease has destroyed the nerves that initiate and transmit pain signals—their behavior is "pathological." If you continue to do something that is clearly not working for you (and may in fact be harmful for you) but hope for—expect or count on—different results, that behavior is pathological. (Some view this as a definition of insanity, which is definitely "pathological" but to the extreme). If you keep engaging in a behavior that makes you feel bad and is, in fact, harmful to your health, while clinging to the belief that it might eventually make you feel good (or perhaps this behavior once upon a time made you feel good but it hasn't for a long, long while), that's "pathological." Or if you accept very short-term relief in exchange for serious side effects and problems, that's pathological.

These behaviors are not "normal"—which is another difficult and confusing word, because after all, what is "normal"? Suppose you are struggling to breathe because you have chronic obstructive pulmonary disease (COPD) and you just can't get enough air into your lungs—that is pathological, or indicative of disease, because "normal" function would be to breathe in and out without effort, with a good exchange of oxygen in and carbon dioxide out, infusing the bloodstream with all the good nutrients and life-giving properties that oxygen supplies and eliminating all the bad stuff (carbon dioxide, toxins) that might have accumulated in your cells and tissues. When your ability to absorb or expel air is impaired, that's pathological, meaning that it suggests or indicates an underlying problem or disease state. Similarly, in a person with diabetes, metabolism of sugar and fat is pathologically impaired, which can cause multiple negative abnormalities and consequences in body functions, such as decreased vision, slowed digestion, and abnormal kidney filtering, to name just a few.

In terms of body functioning, "normal" implies that our organs work the way they are supposed to work. A disease is a pathological or abnormal process that impairs body structure or function, diagnosed by the presence of signs or symptoms. "Pathological" indicates that we are functioning or operating (consciously, subconsciously, or unconsciously) in a dysfunctional way that doesn't support our health and well-being.

Now, on to "pursuit." Why would someone "pursue" a pathological state?

PURSUIT: When we pursue something, we go after it with a desire or need to acquire it—often with an element of desperation. If you are pursuing someone who keeps running away from you, for example, there's a stalker-type quality to the behavior, an obsessiveness to attain what might not be achievable or within reach. So, when we combine "pathological" and "pursuit," we can see that there's a problem.

I once heard a story about an alcoholic Civil War soldier who was trying to explain the depth and breadth of his craving for alcohol. "If there was a bottle of whiskey on the other side of this field," he explained, "and cannons shooting at me from all sides, nothing would stop me from crossing the field to try to reach that bottle." This story shows how "pursuit" is not only obsessive but "pathological" because it would put the soldier in harm's way.

Imagine what this soldier must have been thinking. "Cannon fire everywhere and yet all I can see is that bottle across the field. In fact, that whiskey is more important to me than anything, more essential than life itself. It doesn't seem crazy to me to risk life and limb because that bottle is all I can think about." The soldier's pathological pursuit of alcohol can be seen as a physiological imperative—an intense craving or need. He was unable to think logically and imagine the dire consequences of his actions, for walking across that field would lead to almost certain death. Or worse, perhaps he saw and understood that reality but, because of his pathological craving, he concluded: "I'm going to do it anyway." He was willing to put his very life at risk to reach that bottle and obtain the relief he so desperately needed.

SURVIVAL SALIENCE

My friend and fellow ASAM doctor Kevin McCauley writes about "survival salience," an unconscious mechanism related to a defect in the limbic system, the part of the brain where emotions are linked to behavior and experiences are transformed into memories. In people with this limbic defect, the drug is perceived as essential to survival. That misperception is then transferred to the frontal cortex of the brain where it overrides logic, reason, and judgment. Then and there, an emotional connection is created—one might call it "love" and not be far off—and the addicted person imbues the drug with magical meaning—greater than any natural love you may have known.

Vanessa was a nineteen-year-old heroin addict who told me that at age seventeen, while being anaesthetized with fentanyl before her appendectomy, she experienced a life-changing event. Before she lost consciousness, while counting down from 100, at 98 she decided, "This is the way I want to feel for the rest of my life."

REWARD

The human brain evolved to respond to natural rewards—food, water, sex—because they are essential for health, survival, and reproduction. Opioid drugs (and other addictive drugs including alcohol) activate the same brain reward systems to create "artificial" (but very real) sensations of pleasure, satisfaction, and euphoria. Opioids are also capable of distorting natural reward processes to intensify desire for more drugs (wanting or craving even in the absence of liking the drug's effects), thus causing compulsive drug-seeking and drug-taking behavior. By stimulating and distorting natural reward systems, opioids may generate new brain activities, such as withdrawal states, so that the drug becomes more important than natural rewards that are essential for our survival.

In other words, while the drug's "reward" is similar in nature to the pleasure we get from the first spoonful of a hot fudge sundae, a gulp from a glass of water when we feel as if we're "dying" of thirst, or a lover's caress leading up to the excitement of a sexual encounter, it is significantly more intense. If you take opioid drugs, you may already know all about the reward aspect of these powerful painkillers.

"When I took the Lortabs my doctor prescribed after a skiing acci-dent and knee surgery," Denise, 52, recalls, "I remember exactly what I was thinking. Wow, nobody ever told me it would be like this! I couldn't have imagined this feeling in my wildest dreams! This is abso-lutely fantastic!"

The "instant" rewards faded over time for Denise, just as they did for Sam. "When I take my handful of pills," Sam told me, "I relax, I can tolerate my wife's nagging, I feel a sense of peace wash over me like everything is okay, and I'm fine, better than fine, in fact. If I could live in that feeling, I'd never leave but of course it fades as quickly as it comes on and then I'm left with an awful emptiness and despair. And, of course, the pain comes back. The pain always comes back."

RELIEF

Distinguishing between reward (pleasure) and relief (from pain, anx-iety, fear, depression, and so on) is tricky. The neurological circuitry underlying both reward and relief are inextricably interwoven, and the threads connecting them are particularly intertwined in people living with chronic pain. Imagine for a moment that the attempt to achieve relief is akin to tuning a piano or a guitar string. If you tighten the string too much or if you do not tighten it enough, the instrument is out of balance. When you find the right balance and the tonal quality is pitch perfect, you achieve harmony.

In a similar sense, when you are strung too tight from stress, fear, anger, anxiety, or pain, you find relief when your heart slows down and your muscles relax. If you are chilled because you were caught unpre-pared in a snowstorm on a cold wintry day, you achieve relief when you get home and bundle up in front of a cozy fire. If your blood sugar is low and you feel lightheaded, a glass of orange juice or a handful of raisins will help restore balance. When you're sexually excited and the tension is almost too much to bear, an orgasm brings relief as well as reward. All these experiences offer not just relief from stress and tension but also the rewards of pleasure and comfort.

But for people with chronic pain, and especially for those of us who have become dependent on opioids, the knotted interplay between re-ward and relief gets even tighter and more entangled, as Christopher's story reveals.

CHRISTOPHER'S STORY

▩ Christopher is twenty-three years old. In high school he injured his back in a football game and his doctor prescribed Vicodin.

"Heaven just sort of opened up for me," Christopher told me. "I loved those pills, I couldn't stop thinking about the next dose. But it didn't take long for me to learn about Hell."

When he took Percocet, a more potent opioid prescribed by his doctor, his pain melted away and within days he began to crave the blissful euphoria of those first thirty or forty minutes under the influence of the drug. That's when he felt truly alive and, in his words, "normal." But as the minutes ticked away, the pain came back, and with a vengeance. He gritted his teeth waiting for the next prescribed dose. The rewards (pleasure, euphoria) lasted for only a brief while, diminishing over time, and the relief from pain occurred only at higher and higher doses. After several months, both the rewards and the relief were minimal, yet his body and his brain continued to crave the drugs, if only to experience that evanescent moment of pleasure and relief. Or, in his words, to feel "normal," at least for a little while.

■ ■ ■

Here again, I deeply appreciate my friend Dr. McCauley's approach to describing the hedonic (pleasure) system in our brain that maintains balance around a "pleasure threshold." In other words, our body has a built-in system for regulating pleasure around a hedonic "set point," similar to our body's ability to regulate our temperature to 98.6 degrees. If you have an infection, the brain may alter the set point to, say, 101 or 102 degrees, at which point the immune system kicks into full gear to fight the infection and return the system to normal.

With addiction, the hedonic system is thrown out of whack, causing the set point to get stuck or reprogrammed. The net effect is that the brain becomes anhedonic—it can no longer experience pleasure from experiences that once upon a time offered great comfort, satisfaction, contentment, happiness, joy, or bliss. As Dr. McCauley writes in an essay on the Institute for Addiction Study website:

In essence, the brain is "deaf" to pleasure. The only pleasures it can now sense are VERY "LOUD" pleasures—or those pleasures that cause large fluctuations in dopamine in the limbic structures of the brain. Usually, the things that cause these fluctuations are drugs. If this happens, the limbic (survival) brain is likely to attribute special salience to these drugs as coping mechanisms. Behavior may reorient itself around the drug until the stress is gone.

Now we've got a big problem—the "stress" in addiction is caused and/or magnified by using the drug and even when the drug is withdrawn or no longer available, the stress continues and, in fact, intensifies. Because of this defect that has developed in the addicted person's hedonic system, the drug is imbued with essential, life-giving powers.

I cannot tell you how many times I have heard the phrase, "I need my drugs, I love them more than anything." This is the limbic brain shouting its VERY LOUD message of need. That need shows up as craving, experienced as physical and mental suffering, that creates a physiological imperative—a "survival salience" in Dr. McCauley's words—to use drugs even when these drugs offer few if any rewards and little or no relief as time goes on.

JENNIFER'S STORY

Jennifer Matesa is a writer and author in long-term recovery. Her story of chronic pain, addiction, and recovery brings to life the concepts of "survival salience" and the pathological pursuit of reward manipulated by the limbic brain.

Addiction's obsession and craving don't have clear edges, the way some cancers feel like a pea that you can roll around in the tissue. Obsession and craving are more like tumors that grow in the brain silently, spreading into the cells with invisible tentacles: you discover them only when they've invaded so far that the brain no longer works.

In my midtwenties I sought treatment for migraines and the doctor gave me Stadol, an opioid painkiller. I took it appropriately for a while. Then I began using it for fear, or what doctors call "anxiety." There was a part of my mind that told me I wasn't really abusing it because I still functioned in my life.

The doctor cut me off the third time I asked for an early refill. No conversation about the physical consequences of drug abuse. Instead, rejection, censure—not education.

For a while the doctor gave me Fiorinal (without codeine) and Imitrex, which squeezes the blood vessels to "abort" migraines. When I got pregnant, I had to quit those drugs. In pregnancy I was given Tylenol with Codeine. While pregnant I restricted my intake of any drugs to no more than twice per week. But once my son had weaned, I began taking one or two codeine with my morning tea.

My opioid "high" has always been a boost of energy. I had undiagnosed postpartum depression, and codeine helped me get out of bed and work. My son was a year old, I was consulting and writing a book, and my mother was dying. I had a big house and garden. Now, I think I must have expected myself to have the strength of three women. And my mother had taught me never to ask for help, which reinforced addiction's isolation.

When I began asking for more codeine, my doctor referred me to a headache specialist, who prescribed Vicodin. Then my addiction took off. Hydrocodone, the active ingredient in Vicodin, is four times stronger than codeine. At first, I didn't take a whole tablet, and I didn't take it every day. But soon I was chewing a whole 10-milligram tablet every day with my morning tea. Then the temptation to add another half-tablet was too great to resist. I started running out early, but it worked so well to blunt my pain—and my fear of pain. Thus, craving.

By then my mother had died. I had moved house twice in three years. My body broke down. I had pain everywhere and I was unable to sleep. I cried during the day. For my work I was interviewing pain researchers who were part of the early-2000s push to treat pain with opioid drugs, and they taught me that opioids were so effective for pain because the dose could be raised without limit. So, I took their advice and went to a pain clinic, and that sealed my addiction.

The pain clinic's staff did not ask whether addiction ran in my family. They asked whether I smoked (no), drank (no), or used "recreational drugs." I'd never even smoked a joint. I was a middle-class working mom with chronic pain. They gave me pure hydrocodone. Then they added morphine. Later they switched me to OxyContin, then fentanyl.

For three and a half years I took fentanyl, the strongest full-agonist opioid painkiller known to man. Though I never snorted or injected drugs, I chewed pills, which is inappropriate use. At first I used fentanyl as directed, but later I would cut the 100-microgram fentanyl patches (the equivalent of about 400 to 500 milligrams of morphine per day) into eight pieces and suck on them. The directions instruct patients to stick fentanyl patches on skin, and they warn that excessive heat can lead to fatal overdose. I knew the inside of the mouth is nearly 100 degrees, filled with capillaries that absorb the drug more readily than skin. The drug hit fast. I sometimes could feel my respiration slowing, and there were times at night when I wondered whether I'd be alive in the morning: insanely dangerous and selfish behavior.

Which are two other features of addiction—selfishness, and self-destructive impulses.

By the time I was abusing fentanyl, I was deep into addiction and it was impossible for me to tell my doctor what I was doing. Thus, the final sentinel of addiction: dishonesty, hiding. But early on if a doctor had asked me whether I chewed my pills, I may have been able to admit it—something that might have saved me and the doctors a lot of grief. Physicians need to learn how to screen people for addictive behaviors.

I also knew that my doctor wouldn't have helped me anyway. Her policy was to kick patients who admitted drug abuse into the psychiatric hospital—so I faced not only the prospect of a sudden detox, but also untreated severe pain.

Six years after I'd first gone to the pain clinic, I hired a doctor to detox me. He prescribed Suboxone, containing the semisynthetic opioid buprenorphine, FDA-approved in 2002 for addiction detox and opioid-replacement therapy, also known as "maintenance."

I started on 12 milligrams and tapered quickly to 6. Appetites and senses returned that I hadn't experienced for years: taste and smell; desires for food, sex, work, humor, life. I asked whether I could stay on Suboxone indefinitely. But the DEA allows "sub docs" to treat only a hundred maintenance patients apiece, and he had no empty slots.

Then Suboxone turned on me. My appetites diminished again. I began to obsess about whether I needed to "take something": I was still inside addiction.

What brought me to recovery was admitting I needed even more help. I tapered off Suboxone and put together a community of women in recovery willing to help me. Then I began working out. I cycled and played tennis. I completed two rounds of a fitness program; I started to run. I took action instead of pills. I moved my body, and it healed.

Today I still use the "abortives" [such drugs as Imitrex] for my migraines, and I use a moderate dose of Neurontin for fibromyalgia pain. I meditate. I still have pain, but recovery has taught me that everyone has pain, and I can't get rid of all pain. It has taught me to focus on what I have, instead of what I expect to have, or what I have lost.

■ ■ ■

MAINTENANCE DRUGS—A HOT TOPIC

Jennifer's story of addiction and recovery brings up a timely and controversial topic—maintenance versus abstinence-based treatment. Briefly, for this book is not the place to engage in heated arguments, I need to state that I have grave doubts about the wisdom of using opioid drugs to treat opioid addiction. Suboxone can be very useful in detox and perhaps for the first month of recovery—if the patient is regularly seen and carefully monitored by a qualified health-care professional. But I do not—I cannot, given the horrendous experience of many of my patients—support using Suboxone for years or for life, a treatment regimen some of my addictionist colleagues strongly support.

Medication-assisted treatment (MAT), the current terminology to describe maintenance therapy, is a deeply contentious issue within the medical community. Recently, a doctor who supports the use of maintenance drugs, such as Suboxone and methadone, for long-term use in opioid-addicted patients, announced in a public forum that a physician or treatment center's refusal to use these medications as part of treatment amounts to malpractice. He added that he would go to court to testify against physicians who do not offer these drugs to their patients.

In an attempt to reduce harm—out-of-control use of opioids with all the complications of such use, including overdose and death—many physicians offer such drugs as methadone, which, because it is very long-acting, is less subject to high and low blood levels that occur with such short-acting opioids as Vicodin, Percocet, and Lortab. Suboxone is favored by other physicians because it is thought to have less of an effect on the brain's reward system, thus causing less of a "high." Suboxone is a partial agonist because it fits incompletely into the opiate receptors, causing less of an intoxicating effect and, like methadone, it is also long-acting. The drug's other unique characteristic is that it binds tightly to the receptor, basically closing the door to other opioid drugs, and thus it is thought to reduce craving.

Like all other opioids, both methadone and Suboxone work on opioid receptor sites and alter the brain—of that we are certain. What remains to be seen is to what extent and effect this occurs.

The debate over medication-assisted treatment will continue for many years and the final decision about whether to use drugs like Suboxone or methadone in the long term is yours and yours alone. But I do need to repeat once again that I do not support the use of potentially habit-forming and addictive drugs to treat people who are addicted to or dependent upon drugs. Both Suboxone and methadone definitely cause significant physical dependence and you will most likely have difficulty cutting back or stopping these drugs once you start because of withdrawal. Furthermore, the possibilities for reigniting the underlying addiction are real and obvious, not to mention the potentially harmful side effects of maintenance drugs and the extreme difficulties when stopping them.

For completeness, I should mention naltrexone, another medication that blocks the opioid receptor, competing with any opioid that may be taken. (Incidentally, naltrexone also decreases craving for alcohol and is marketed for that effect.) Naltrexone comes in several forms: an oral medication, an injectable formulation (Vivitrol) that lasts about a month, and an implant placed under the patient's skin that lasts six to twelve months. Patients who use naltrexone do not experience the pleasure or pain-relieving effects if they take opioids and thus they tend to use them less or not at all. While there is no clear evidence of the effect of naltrexone on pain, some of my colleagues believe the drug has the beneficial effect of reducing pain as well as diminishing relapse to opioid drugs and alcohol.

In Chapters 6–10 I will offer a variety of tools and techniques that work to relieve pain and overcome addiction. For many people, these strategies work wonders. Holistic approaches (those focusing on the whole person rather than the malady or disease) to treatment and re- covery from chronic pain are both safe and effective. Furthermore, they put you in charge of your own recovery. My ultimate goal is to empower you to make the choices that will improve the quality of your life.

DEPENDENCE OR ADDICTION?

Let's come back to the perplexing question that patients and their family members often ask, usually with a great deal of fear: "Am I de- pendent on drugs or am I addicted to them?" The difference between addiction and dependence is not easy to tease apart. This discussion may get a little complicated, but most people find that understanding the neurological and biochemical nature of dependence and addiction allows them to develop insight into whichever diagnosis fits best. And by doing so, they are able to create a firm and solid foundation for long- term recovery.

What is dependence? Basically, it's the brain's and body's demand— experienced as "need"—to take the drugs to avoid uncomfortable and often painful withdrawal symptoms. Your brain has adapted its func- tioning to accommodate to these chemicals, and when the levels circu- lating through the brain and body drop, you suffer. (Long-term opioid use also has the additional potential effect of altering your natural pain- killers and lessening their effectiveness.) So, you feel a need to get the drugs back into your body and that need can be overpowering. Once the drugs are completely out of your system—a withdrawal process that can be uncomfortable and painful—you won't experience craving and compulsion to use. That is, *if* you are dependent and not addicted.

If you are addicted, however, you will most likely experience crav- ing and compulsion to use even months, years, or decades after the drugs are no longer in your system. Why? For a majority of addicted in- dividuals, the reward pathways were "abnormal" before drugs were ever taken. You may have inherited a multitude of genes passed down from one generation to another that influence and enhance the rewards you experience when you use alcohol or other drugs. In other words, your brain gets a significant pleasurable jolt from taking the drugs, and when the drugs wear off, you find yourself wanting, craving, needing—and finding a way to acquire—more.

Over time as your brain adapts its functioning, the drugs don't give you the same relief and reward because you have developed tolerance—you need a higher dose of the drug to achieve the same level of response—so you increase the dose. If you successfully stop the drugs—*if you are dependent*—you will not experience a craving to use again. If you are addicted, however, the craving will surface, sometimes when you least expect it, despite the fact that you no longer have the drugs in your system. Cravings may continue for months and even years and are one of the major causes of relapse.

For people with chronic pain, craving typically presents in the form of pain. Claire, for example, was addicted to multiple drugs when she came to treatment. "For me, the experience of having pain was always and is still always associated with craving a drug to gain relief," she said. "Will that ever go away, Doc?" Six years later, she continues to have periodic flare-ups of pain, accompanied by cravings for relief, but she has not relapsed and is more accustomed to these compulsive urges.

Genes are only part of the story of how addiction develops for some people. Environmental stressors can also alter the normal reward system pathways. If you experienced trauma or abuse as a child, you may be more susceptible to addiction because of the interplay between your emotions and your physiological responses. You may experience a hypersensitive response to stressful situations, and your ability to "self-soothe" may be impaired. The circumstances surrounding your initial drug use will also play a role in your susceptibility to addiction. If you are first exposed to addictive drugs in your teens, for example, you are much more likely to become addicted because your brain is still developing and therefore more vulnerable to the effects of these drugs (e.g., nicotine, alcohol, cannabis, opioids, sedatives, and others).

So, in summary: *Addiction is dependence plus.* If you are dependent on opioid drugs, you will not experience craving months or years after you stop using them; but if you are addicted, your reward system can be triggered at any time (more frequently in early recovery) by people, places, or cues that remind you of the extreme and extraordinary pleasure you experienced when you took drugs. These unwelcome and unconscious pinpricks of pleasant memories related to drug use underlie the experience of craving, which may lead to an uncontrollable urge to use drugs. Cravings are not always or even usually overpowering and can, in fact, be subtle and tricky. Sometimes they come in dreams or as casual benign thoughts that seem to just pop up as we go about our day.

The following questionnaire may be helpful to you (and to your family members) in determining whether you are addicted to the medications you take to relieve your chronic pain. Family members also find this questionnaire helpful as they seek to understand whether a loved one's drug use is spiraling out of control.

Am I Addicted to My Pain Medication?
A Self-Test

—— 1. Have you ever taken more of your medications or taken them more frequently than was prescribed?

—— 2. Have you ever used another doctor because your doctor wouldn't prescribe any more medication or increase your dosage?

—— 3. Do you find yourself looking at the clock to find out when you can take your next dose of medication?

—— 4. Have you used alcohol while taking prescriptions, to enhance the medications' effect, even knowing you were not supposed to?

—— 5. Have you ever used illegal drugs while taking prescribed medications?

—— 6. Do you have more than one doctor who is prescribing medications for you? If the answer is yes, are those doctors aware of all the medications you are taking?

—— 7. Have you ever gone to an emergency room to get additional medications because the ones you had were not enough?

—— 8. Have you ever run out of a prescription before you were supposed to because you used more than was prescribed?

—— 9. Did you ever think "as needed" meant you could use as much as you wanted to, when you wanted to?

—— 10. Have you ever lied to a doctor about why you needed another prescription filled?

—— 11. Have you ever exaggerated your reported pain level just in case you had more pain later or to get another or a stronger prescription?

continues

continued

—— 12. Did you have addiction problems before your chronic pain?

—— 13. Have you ever thought, "I can't live without medication"?

—— 14. Have you ever gotten a prescription and lied to your spouse or other family members or friends about it?

—— 15. Have you ever lied to your family members, friends, employers, or others about how much medication you are taking?

—— 16. Are you taking prescription medication and supplementing it with over-the-counter medication?

—— 17. Are you taking other prescriptions to deal with the side effects of your pain medication (e.g., sleep aids, stimulants, anti-anxiety drugs, or the mood-altering muscle relaxant Soma)?

—— 18. Have you ever taken anyone else's pain medication?

—— 19. Have you ever stolen, forged, or altered a prescription, or called in a prescription by impersonating medical staff?

—— 20. Have you ever crushed, snorted, or injected your medication or taken it in a way other than the way it was intended to be taken?

—— 21. Have you ever overdosed or needed medical help because you took too much medication?

—— 22. Have you ever experienced a blackout (memory loss) caused by medication?

—— 23. Have you experienced legal consequences as a result of taking your medication, such as a DUI?

—— 24. Have you had a friend, spouse, or family member express concern regarding your use of pain medication?

—— 25. Have you ever taken pain medications to deal with other issues such as stress or anxiety?

None of these questions necessarily defines addiction, but if you answered yes to any of these, you should not rule out the possibility of addiction. The more "yes" answers you have, the greater the cause for concern about addiction.

Important Note: Do not use this test to judge yourself negatively; use it as part of a process of learning and examining that is necessary for success in pain recovery.

COMPLEX DEPENDENCE

Things are not neat and tidy in the addiction world. When chronic pain and addiction to opioid drugs enter the picture, we're dealing with two stigmatized illnesses ("She's always complaining about her pain." "Why doesn't he just quit taking those drugs if they're not working?"). Both chronic pain and addiction are generated in the brain and, through unconscious processes, impact behavior in profound ways . . . they twist and contort emotions . . . they compel us to isolate ourselves from people and experiences we love the most . . . and they feed on each other so that a small spark turns into a raging fire, which ultimately becomes a death-dealing inferno.

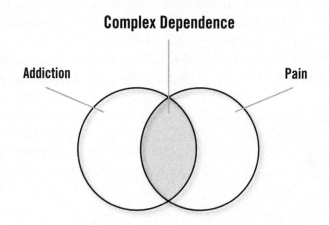

And then there's this middle ground where people are definitely dependent on opioid drugs to relieve their chronic pain, and somewhere along the line (whether from that very first pill or many years and doses later), some subtle, unseen part of the brain is stimulated to pathologically pursue reward as well as to pursue relief. When this happens, we typically feel good when we take the drugs, we continue to take the drugs as prescribed—for example, we aren't likely to snort or chew or hoard or steal or sell or buy them from drug dealers—and we don't experience that LOUD voice in our brains that tells us to get more, more, more.

But—in such cases we simply can't draw a clear definitive boundary between addiction and dependence. The boundaries between pathological and non-pathological pursuit are blurred by what is termed complex, or iatrogenic, dependence. When you take an extra Lortab because your pain has not totally gone away with the prescribed dose and then you run out of your prescription a few days before you can renew it ("Why didn't the doctor give me more when my pain is so bad?") . . . when you "borrow" a few Vicodins from your husband's prescription that has been sitting in the medicine cabinet for three months after his shoulder surgery ("After all, he doesn't need them anymore") . . . when you take the drug before the pain occurs, in anticipation, to prevent the pain ("I know it's coming and I don't want to feel it") . . . when you take your daughter's pain pills left over from her dental surgery and find yourself wondering, ("Why in the world didn't she use them all; how bizarre is that?") . . . are you really pursuing pain relief or is there something that's not quite right (pathological) about your use?

Well, in a very real sense there is something not quite right about that situation, for (1) you are breaking the rules of the agreement you had with your doctor; (2) you are taking pills prescribed for someone else (this is against the law, even if the person gives you permission); (3) you are using defense mechanisms, such as *rationalizing* ("I'm in pain" or "I know I will be soon and I want to prevent it from happening"); *justifying* ("I wasn't stealing from my neighbor or buying pills from a drug dealer"); *minimizing* ("I only took three extra pills"); and *blaming* ("The doctor should have given me more").

Does your complex dependence on the drugs put you into the middle section of the Venn diagram or have you already crossed the line into addiction? I don't know. I wish I did. A dentist patient of mine asked me recently whether his drug use had evolved into drug dependence or, possibly, addiction. He was in severe pain from spinal stenosis—the open spaces in his spine had narrowed due to arthritic changes, putting pressure on his nerves and causing intense pain, numbness, muscle weakness, and both bowel and bladder problems. He took his pills as his doctor prescribed, but every once in a while he'd ask a friend to give him a few extras. Then, one fateful day, when he was in a lot of "really *really* bad" pain and had a full schedule of patients stacked up in fifteen-minute intervals, he asked his assistant to inject him with Demerol from the office stock.

When he told me this story and asked whether I thought he might have a drug problem, I leveled with him, expressing my deep concern that his "problem" might in fact be opioid addiction. He resisted that diagnosis, despite the red flags flying all over the place, and refused the offer of treatment. Soon enough, however, the decision about whether his drug use was "pathological" was taken out of his hands when his assistant reported the Demerol incident to his partner, who notified the state dental board, and he was forced to seek treatment for addiction or lose his license to practice dentistry.

It used to be that I would go to the mats over this issue, wrestling and tangling with patients in an attempt to help them see and understand that their drug use is problematic. I've tried the "You've got a problem, you better do something about it right now" approach, and that judgmental, clinical attitude alienated many more people than it helped. I've also tried: "How can you do this to your family?" and learned that guilt and shame are prevalent feelings for people wrestling with their drug use and that inducing more of these emotions merely pushes them away. I've learned that it doesn't pay to fight because ultimately, the only person who can decide if regular opioid use has morphed into dependence on drugs or if dependence has crossed the line into addiction is you.

Only you can honestly and sincerely determine whether opioid drugs have become a serious and perhaps even a life-threatening problem for you. A patient once asked me for a blood test "to find out once and for all whether or not I have addiction," and I had to tell her that, unfortunately, we do not have conclusive diagnostic tests for addiction. I wish we did—and I believe that someday we will.

In the meantime, I find that the list of behaviors in the following chart can be helpful when a patient (or a family member) wonders about the possibility of addiction.

DEPENDENCE OR ADDICTION: WHY DOES IT MATTER?

The important question is, can you safely take opioid drugs to treat your pain? That's the real issue here. That's what is at stake. If you are addicted, you can't. For someone with complex dependence, I am less certain. Ask yourself: Can I continue to take opioids successfully—in

92

12 Behaviors That Might Signify an Addiction Problem

1. **Running out early:** You run out of pills before your scheduled refill. Often this means that you have to "tough it out" for a few days (or weeks) because you doubled or tripled the dose and can't get a refill.
2. **Prescriptions from multiple physicians:** One client I worked with had prescriptions for addictive drugs from six different prescribers: her surgeon, orthopedic surgeon, two general practitioners, a pain doctor, and a dentist.
3. **Forceful, sometimes belligerent requests** for additional prescriptions, stronger medications, or higher dosages.
4. **Snorting or chewing pills, sucking on patches:** You use the pills that have been prescribed for you, but you don't use them as instructed ("take one tablet nightly," or "take one tablet in the morning and one before bedtime").
5. **Using illicit drugs:** You supplement your normal prescription regimen with alcohol, illicit drugs (cocaine, marijuana), or extra pills from a different doctor or that you obtain from someone else.
6. **Regularly losing prescriptions:** "The dog ate the prescription." "It fell into the toilet and got flushed down the drain." "My wife mistakenly tossed it in the garbage with the newspaper."
7. **Using the drugs for purposes other than intended:** After a fight with your spouse, you take an extra Vicodin because you're feeling angry and anxious. Or you have a stressful meeting in a few hours and decide to take an extra Oxy to calm your nerves. Or you take your Lortabs to get going in the morning.
8. **Asking for specific drugs in specific dosages:** "Those Oxy 60s just aren't hitting the pain, would you prescribe Oxy 100s instead?" "If you would write me a prescription for 4 mg Dilaudid, I think that would do the trick."
9. **Selling a prescription to pay for other drugs:** You sell all but five of the Suboxone you got from the doctor to buy some black tar heroin from your dealer, saving the five pills in case you run out of heroin.

continues

continued

10. **Obtaining prescription drugs from non-medical people:** One patient bought 120 OxyContins from an elderly neighbor who had cancer (the neighbor sold the drugs to pay his rent).

11. **Prescription forgery:** Calling in prescriptions to the pharmacy; forging prescriptions on pads produced on your computer or stolen from your doctor's office; changing the number of pills on the prescription.

12. **Ignoring family members' concerns:** Your spouse, children, or parents tell you they're worried about your drug use. You shrug off their concerns or lash out in anger, telling them to mind their own business; or you find a way to blame them ("You're always on my back." "You have no idea how much pain I am in." "Why should I have to answer to you, you're not my doctor!").

other words, are the drugs working to reduce my pain, and more important, to improve my life (or, at the very least, not diminish my quality of life)?

If you decide to use opioids, please pay *close attention* to your response, especially your level of function. Track this carefully over time. Get input from concerned friends and family, because you may not be able to rely on your own perceptions to assess accurately how you are reacting and behaving. (So often, families see what is happening long before you can.) And if you stop and the cycle starts up again—escalating doses with decreasing benefits—then I'd say you have definitively proven that opioids are not for you. It may or may not be addiction, but if you have a history of complex dependence even with no evidence of addiction, it is highly likely that opioids are not the solution.

Sleeping pills and anti-anxiety medications are also not the solution. In a well-meaning attempt to help you get a good night's sleep and/or to relieve anxiety, your doctor may prescribe these medications. While the drugs may help for a while, their long-term dangers are serious and potentially deadly. Combining these drugs with narcotic painkillers increases the dangers of dependence and addiction, worsens the side effects associated with each drug, and all too often results in accidental overdose and death.

To help you understand complex dependence, I'd like you to meet Alice. Her story is adapted with her permission from a book she is writing titled *The Healthiest You Can Be*.

ALICE'S STORY

Alice suffered severe, life-threatening injuries in a boating accident in the Caribbean when she fell while waterskiing and the motorboat ran over her, shredding her left buttock, most of her thigh, and almost severing her leg.

"I don't remember much about the trip to the hospital. I do remember arriving, because that is when the agony finally started. I was given a morphine drip to help dull the pain, but it was still excruciating. I had lost a huge amount of blood and could hear the medical staff discussing the fact that I was unlikely to make it as they couldn't get enough blood on the island to replace all the liters I had lost and was continuing to lose."

Alice's leg became badly infected and she was transferred to a hospital in Miami, Florida, where she spent two months as the medical staff battled to keep the infection under control. She then flew back to her home in England where doctors tried to save her leg.

"The doctors reopened the leg and used stem cells and donor bone, both from my own pelvis and from a deceased donor, to start building a new scaffold around which my leg would hopefully regenerate healthy tissue. Between the original injury and all the tissue that had been removed to keep the infection under control, I had very little leg left. I had to lie very still for fourteen months to allow the rebuilt leg to start healing before I could even contemplate starting to use it again.

"I am not sure whether or not I was offered any psychological treatment at this point; my impression is that possibly I was offered counselling and turned it down. Early on I suffered from post-traumatic stress syndrome and had a number of terrible flashbacks, at which stage I had some emergency psychiatric help and had been offered some medication that I didn't want to take. I had never dealt with the trauma and felt a great need to gain some control over my life. The last thing I wanted to do was to rake over my experience of the accident and the emotions I had felt in the immediate aftermath . . .

"Now, I can see very clearly that I was in great denial about the emotional journey that lay ahead. I focused relentlessly on how to get better, which was a good thing in many ways, but neglected to consider the reality, which was that it was going to be a long, hard struggle, and that life might never be the same again. I suppressed feelings of anger and distress so deeply that even I was largely unaware of them."

■ ■ ■

Alice was twenty-two when she had her accident. I met her twelve years later and the word *adorable* immediately came to mind. A tiny woman, not quite five feet tall and weighing barely 100 pounds, she leaned forward in her chair, eyes wide open, attentive, listening, eager to learn everything she could, believing that even if the pain diminished a little bit, all the work she invested would be worth it. When I looked at the long list of drugs she was taking and the incredibly high dosages of those drugs, I simply couldn't believe that she was able to walk, talk, think, react. Using a morphine equivalent calculator, I estimated that the fentanyl (patches and sublingual doses), Percocet, and OxyContin she'd been taking as prescribed by her doctors was the equivalent of 22,000 mg of morphine each day—220 times the dosage doctors consider "safe."

Alice's detox alone took almost three weeks and she was miserable through much of it. How she maintained her positive attitude and endured the torture of coming off such high doses of drugs, in spite of everything we could do to keep her comfortable and reduce her pain, I will never know. She was always a cheerful force in the community, avidly practicing yoga, meditating, and enthusiastically participating in group activities. She rarely complained, but during our talks she often expressed understandable frustration with her limitations—the limp she would have for the rest of her life, her fear that she might never have children, the slow pace of her exercise routines, and the pain, pain, pain. My heart broke for her.

Alice stayed in the pain program for five more weeks after detox and improved significantly over time. Her pain levels dropped a little, she slept better despite the troublesome and often high levels of pain, and she was able to eliminate all medications except for a low dose of tramadol. Tramadol is an interesting drug. Biochemically, it is not an opioid and most physicians believe it is safe and non-addictive—even though it works in the body just like an opioid, it can be habit-forming, and at high doses it can cause seizures. In short, it is not a benign drug, and I had concerns about prescribing it for Alice, just as she worried about the drug's effect on her life. I'll never forget the expression of deep concern on her face when she told me that she never wanted to go back to the state of numbness and disconnection from life that she experienced when she was "doped up" on opioid drugs.

But we had to do something because she simply could not manage the pain without medication. No one could manage that level of pain without some kind of relief. I was certain that she wasn't addicted—she had taken the incredibly high doses of medications exactly as prescribed by her doctors, she did not have an intense craving to use (and, in fact, she was highly motivated to get off all opioid drugs), and her use was never characterized by a pathological pursuit of pleasure or relief. She definitely had complex dependence, with a truly horrific underlying structural cause of her pain, and she needed some measure of relief. I believed that tramadol would be relatively safe for her, but because the drug had the potential to be habit-forming and cause tolerance and physical dependence, I had some nagging concerns.

Alice returned to England after eight weeks in treatment and she e-mails me periodically to let me know that she is continuing on the steady dose of tramadol and able to tolerate the pain. With her characteristic energy and exuberance, she meditates and practices yoga daily and now works as a psychologist with a focus on integrative medicine, writing her book in her spare time. She inspires me and everyone who meets her.

I cannot end her story, however, on a "happily ever after" note. Alice still has a high pain level at times, and while the low dose of tramadol helps, it does not erase the pain. In a recent e-mail Alice confessed that she was having "one of my bad days when you are just desperate for something strong to take the pain away."

What should she do? What should I do, how can I help her? That's the question that keeps me up at night. I strongly believe that when patients pay close attention to the emotional work—as well as the physical, mental, and spiritual strategies I will describe in Part 2—they will get better. I know from my own experience and from witnessing the recoveries of hundreds of patients who commit themselves to "doing the work," that if you are willing and if you put in the effort, you will have better results. Willingness + effort = good results.

But what about people like Alice—people like you, perhaps—who have the willingness and devote consistent, daily effort but continue to experience unrelenting, intractable pain? Patients with complex dependence are my most challenging. Do I ask you to "bear with it" and prescribe non-narcotic drugs, hoping that the pain is, indeed, bearable and will fade over time—or do I write a prescription for stronger drugs or higher dosages, thereby consigning you to a diminished quality of life, blunted mood and emotions, and the possibility of pushing you closer to addiction?

In her e-mail, Alice went on to state that she knows opioids are only "a temporary solution that will make things worse . . . I am not sure where I would be now if I hadn't been through the treatment program, which has totally changed my life. I have my freedom back again and that is priceless."

Alice's story may very well be your story, too—not in its specifics but in the knowledge, gained by experience, that freedom is hard won. Freedom—from pain, from suffering, from dependence on addictive drugs—is paradoxical, for all of us living with chronic pain will experience "bad" days when we crave instant, blessed relief from extreme discomfort. I wish I had an answer, a magical cure. But I don't. And so I try to mirror Alice's strength, having faith that she will continue to make it through the rough patches with her characteristic courage and grace. I trust her statement that freedom is priceless. And I know in my heart that she is right.

If you're unsure about the difference between dependence and addiction, take a look at the following chart.

A FINAL WORD ABOUT
DEFENSE MECHANISMS

Defense mechanisms are part of our human existence. What we are defending is often hard to identify. We are, in essence, protecting what we perceive as important to our survival. Perhaps we protect ourselves

If you have DEPENDENCE	If you have ADDICTION
Pain is relieved or manageable with medications. My pain is greatly relieved with medication. I definitely need the drugs to help me deal with the pain and sometimes I can manage with non-narcotic drugs.	**No appreciable decrease in pain with medications** At first the drugs worked better than I ever anticipated. But over time, the pain came back and the pills stopped working. Now I'm in more pain than ever.
No significant changes in functioning due to medication I'm still able to function well while I'm taking the drugs—even though I still have pain. In fact, the drugs allow me to function better because the pain decreases.	**Significant decrease in functioning due to medication** I'm having trouble concentrating, I can't sleep, I'm constipated, I feel depressed and irritable, and I spend a lot of time in bed.
No significant effect on relationships; family members are not concerned regarding use The pills I take for pain have not affected my relationships with the people I love. In fact, I feel like I am more loving because I have less pain.	**Ongoing relationship problems and concerns from family regarding use** My drug use has had a serious impact on my marriage and my ability to be a loving, attentive parent.
Able to work with no significant decrease in job performance Even though I continue to take drugs for pain, I am able to concentrate, focus on my work and show up regularly.	**Unable to work or significant impairment due to medication** I just can't be bothered with deadlines. My memory isn't what it used to be. The pain and the drugs interfere with my ability to work. I frequently call in sick.
Stable or maintenance dose of pain medication I'm on an intermittent dose of painkillers, and the dosage hasn't changed over the years.	**Steadily increasing dose and frequency of medications, with little or no decrease in pain** I need more and more of the drug—higher doses, stronger drugs—and yet the pain keeps getting worse.

continues

continued

If you have DEPENDENCE	If you have ADDICTION
Emotional stability and acceptance of any physical limitations I experience normal ups and downs, but overall I'm emotionally stable and I accept the fact that I have to live with some measure of pain and disability.	**Emotional instability and increasing lack of acceptance regarding physical limitations** I am bitter and angry one minute and suicidal the next. I can barely walk because I am in so much pain. The drugs just aren't cutting it for me, but I can't imagine life without them.
No significant cognitive impairment due to medication use I can think clearly on the medications I am taking, even though the pain is still there.	**Significant cognitive impairment due to use (foggy thinking, difficulty concentrating, memory problems)** When I use the opioids—always as prescribed by my doctor—my mind simply does not work. I can't write, think, talk, or remember important details.
Using medications only for pain relief I use the drugs only for pain relief; they do not have a significant beneficial psychological or emotional effect on me.	**Relying on medications for emotional effect** I take the drugs to help me deal with stress, anxiety, depression, and anger. They really don't help me cope with the grief I feel over losing the life I once had, but at least I can escape for a while.

from being hurt by others—pushing them away before they can hurt us. We may defend behaviors such as taking drugs or staying in bed all day as if our life depends on them—even when they are really doing us harm. We might utilize defense mechanisms such as denial, rationalization, justification, minimization, and blaming in all kinds of situations and for all sorts of reasons. "I don't have a drug problem since I take the drugs as prescribed." "I don't want to go to the doctor, the pain will go away." "I wouldn't be falling asleep if you talked about interesting stuff instead of your work."

Being able to see and acknowledge your defense mechanisms is not easy. In fact, this is really tough work. But you are reading this book because you know something has to change and defense mechanisms stand in the way of progress. Understanding why you have erected them is essential, even if dismantling them is not in any sense simple or effortless.

It may help to think of defense mechanisms as curtains that we draw across our lives because we feel vulnerable or insecure. Often we fear judgment or censure. We can hide behind our defenses for a while, tend to our wounds, gather our strength, and then pull the curtains aside when we feel ready to move forward by accepting responsibility, forgiving ourselves or others, or making changes in our life.

But with addiction something different happens. We draw the curtains around our life with regularity and great emotional intensity. We don't just shut people out for a few minutes while we retreat in embarrassment or shame—instead, we close ourselves off for hours, days, months, years. We *hide*, for addiction is all about hiding, and defense mechanisms help us shut out the people, situations, and experiences that threaten us. And we hide from ourselves; we avoid seeing the truth, at all costs. To put it more bluntly, we shut the curtain on anything and everything that might threaten our ability to keep using the drugs that our brain has come to need and that our body (brain) craves.

Remember, if you are addicted, you do not have control over this craving—it is unconscious mental and physical desire generated deep within the limbic brain that drives you to use, no matter how strong-willed, kind-hearted, mature, and responsible you might be. Your very survival, your brain tells you, depends on getting the drug(s) into your body and quieting that deep, undeniable need or drive. Your brain has been hijacked, and your frontal cortex is no longer in charge.

I was working in addiction treatment before I got sober and sometimes, when describing a blackout or a problematic behavior to patients, I would hear a voice in my head saying, "You do that." It was mostly a whisper, and I was quick to shut it up because my defense mechanisms allowed me to shout down the truth so that I could keep using the drugs. If I let down my guard and permitted myself to see the truth, I would have to *do* something (such as stop using, perish the thought). At that point, I wasn't ready because I couldn't conceive of life without the drugs. How could I relax, sleep, wake up, and manage my physical and emotional pain?

Those of us who deny, rationalize, justify, minimize, and blame of-ten seem perfectly logical in our arguments. It can be really hard to tell the difference between a defense mechanism and the truth. This is one reason family members often feel as if they are the ones who are going crazy—when they express their concern to their addicted loved one, the arguments thrown back at them actually seem to make sense.

Here's a "logical" argument often used by people in chronic pain—maybe you've used it yourself: "If I wasn't in pain, do you think I'd be taking these drugs?" The only way to prove whether this is true is to take your pain away (which, of course, is impossible) and then see whether you stop using drugs. In the absence of this kind of proof, all we have is our own individual subjective experience of what happens to us when we take the drug(s).

If you have chronic pain and opioid addiction, you are truly between a rock and a hard place—because you take the pills for pain (even if you take them exactly as your doctor prescribed) and the pills diminish your pain (even if you have to take higher and higher doses over time or switch to stronger drugs), who can argue with you that the pills aren't working? They do work and because they work (at least for a time) so quickly and effectively, you are loath to give them up. You have be-come attached to them, convinced that you need them and cannot live without them.

Over time and with effective treatment, most patients come to re-alize that they took opioids for two primary reasons: (1) for relief of physical pain and (2) to feel better emotionally. "I thought I was only taking the Lortabs for pain," one patient told me, "but then I realized I got energy from my Lortabs. I was attached to them. I got more from the pills than I ever realized or could admit. And there was something not-quite-right about that." That statement marked the beginning of this patient's recovery.

For most people, the impetus to seek help comes from outside (others) rather than inside (self). Paul, whose story we tell in Chapter 2, didn't go to treatment because he suddenly saw the light but rather because he felt the heat.

I lived in fear of the pain and what it was going to do next. I lived in fear of intervention mainly from the medical licensure board, which did ultimately happen, and I certainly lived in fear of running out of pain pills. I then developed a very short fuse and was very quick to anger with minimal reasons. As it progressed, the anger became increasingly more intense and sustained, with a great deal of it directed at those closest to me who I loved the most. With all of this came self-imposed isolation. I continued to withdraw from everyone and everything, culminating in my isolation from God and feeling utterly alone in my suffering. I knew death was coming and I was perfectly fine with that fact. I had lost all hope that my pain and suffering would ever stop.

I well remember the feeling after the investigator from the Board delivered the summons in person for me to appear for a meeting with the evaluation committee. I sat down behind my desk and when the panic and nausea resolved I simply thought, "Well, it's finally happened and I'm still alive." I actually felt relief at some level. Without this specific intervention in this way at this time, I likely would have died from an unintentional overdose and never made it into treatment.

Treatment saved Paul's life. Unfortunately, not everyone can afford inpatient treatment, and insurance plans often cover just a fraction of the cost (or none at all). What can you do if you have limited financial resources and treatment is not available to you?

In Part 2 you will find a multitude of techniques and strategies that you can learn on your own, in your own home, to help relieve your pain and regain your enthusiastic participation in life's everyday activities. These are the strategies we teach our patients and there is just one absolute requirement for them to work—commitment. You *must* commit yourself heart and soul to this program of recovery. You must do the work. Half-hearted attempts will not work. Throw yourself into this program and have faith that it will work. Because it will, if you work at it. I promise you that.

Part 2

OVERCOMING

The most authentic thing about us is our
capacity to create, to overcome, to endure, to transform,
to love and to be greater than our suffering.

—BEN OKRI, NIGERIAN POET AND NOVELIST

Pain, as we have emphasized, is part of life. It cannot successfully be avoided or eliminated. The question is: What do we do with our pain? In Part 2 you will learn about the power of your mind to redirect beliefs and "unthink" destructive thoughts. You will discover how to restore physical balance through exercise, sleep, acupressure, and both traditional and alternative healing methods. And you will find ways to balance your emotional and spiritual health with step-by-step strategies encouraging mindfulness, gratitude, acceptance, forgiveness, and reconnection to others and the world around you.

FIVE

DISCOVERING THE POWER OF THE MIND

Challenging Assumptions and Achieving Realistic Expectations

As a single footstep will not make a path on the earth,
so a single thought will not make a pathway in the mind.
To make a deep physical path, we walk again and again.
To make a deep mental path, we must think over and
over the kind of thoughts we wish to dominate our lives.

—HENRY DAVID THOREAU

The antidote to the physical problems that plague you can be found in the power of your mind. With careful attention and growing awareness, you can use your mind to challenge old destructive thought patterns and create new ways of coping with difficult, seemingly insurmountable obstacles.

To accomplish this challenging work, you will need to develop a willingness to do the following:

- Suspend disbelief.
- Be openhearted, gentle, and patient with yourself and others.
- Be courageous.
- Be diligent.

In my first meeting with a patient, I emphasize the critical importance of these four "keys" to success in treatment and beyond. I'll never forget my very first conversation with Harriet. Although she was just twenty-nine years old, her face was lined with the wrinkles of a sixty-year-old. She had a running "script" about how "this can't work."

"I will end up homeless, because my family won't let me return if I don't complete treatment."

"My pain will be 'off the charts' and you won't give me anything to treat it. I'll just be flopping around in bed like a fish, miserable and writhing in agony."

"I can't sleep without my Ambien; at least knock me out for this next week, or better yet, just shoot me now!"

Harriet had a flair for the dramatic, that's for sure, but I knew that her rapid-fire speech pattern was generated by her distorted perceptions of life and, of course, by her narrative about her pain that arose out of these visions of hell that her mind conjured up. She was jumpy because in addition to withdrawing from opioids (Vicodin and fentanyl), benzodiazepines (Valium), and sedatives (Ambien), she had been using methamphetamine daily for the week before she came into treatment. Her thoughts were being filtered through a brain that was chemically overstimulated. And the litany of words that poured out told a story that reverberated in her mind, a virtual picture book detailing the moment-by-moment catastrophes that awaited her.

"My mind is like a pinball machine," she said. "Can you picture the spring going back and popping the ball into the chute—rounding the bend and . . . *bounce?* . . ."

Yes, I could picture it. I haven't used drugs of any kind for quite a while, but believe me, meth addicts aren't the only ones with "monkey minds," as Buddhists call it. My thoughts also bounce around at times like a pinball machine. Work . . . meetings, patient needs, lecture to give at four . . . *bounce* . . . presentation to give next month . . . did I make my reservations for Atlanta . . . plane crash in the Ukraine . . . so tragic . . . *bounce* . . . there's always turbulence flying into Las Vegas, especially in the summer . . . *bounce* . . . I have to pay the electric bill today . . . *bounce* . . . I wonder how Laura and John are, I'm looking forward to dinner with them, where should we eat? . . . *bounce, bounce* . . . I have a Groupon that's gonna expire . . . *bounce* . . . I have to take my car in, the tires are low again, why is that? . . . *bounce* . . . I miss my folks . . . I miss Denny . . . What's for dinner tonight? . . . *bounce, bounce, bounce.*

Bells are ringing all over the place as the ball bounces from place to place in the pinball machine that is my mind, generating thought after thought, fragment after fragment. And that was just the last sixty seconds of my inner dialogue.

THE POWER TO CHANGE

Tackling the painful and destructive inner dialogues that prattle on 24/7 in your mind and redirecting your beliefs and theories about who you are and what purpose you have on this earth are essential before you can embark on any of the remaining steps and strategies in Part 2. You need to understand and fully absorb the fact that you have the wherewithal and the power to change those dialogues, or better yet, shut them off completely. If you accept this important truth and do the work, *your pain will decrease and you will have a better life!* So, right here and right now I ask you to make a commitment to do the work outlined in the rest of this book.

Listening to Harriet, I quickly picked up on her deprecating self-talk, the nonstop chatter that would sabotage her chances of getting better. I challenged her—and I challenge you—to simply stop the tape that says, "This can't work." It will start up as often as once every few seconds, so you will have to keep saying, "Stop." Say it gently to yourself over and over, again and again, as if you were training a recalcitrant puppy ("Stay . . . stay . . . good! Oops . . . stay . . . stay"). No smacking the pup, and likewise, no beating up on yourself when you don't do this perfectly. Eventually, with practice, the volume of the message will turn down a notch or two. Some of the messages that need to stop are:

"My pain will never ever go away!"
"I'm going to end up in a wheelchair!"
"I'm lazy and unmotivated, and I deserve to be in pain!"
"My family is going to desert me; it's inevitable; how can they put up with me?"
"I'm just like my mother, a chronic complainer!"

You will also need to be realistic about your expectations and remind yourself that you cannot and will not find instant, magical relief in these pages. The only thing that offers instant relief is a drug, an effect that is only temporary and, as we have seen, all too often backfires in the long run. Change requires time, commitment, dedication, and a healthy dose of faith in your body's self-healing powers. Believing can truly make it so.

Many people I work with question their ability to recover and, at the same time, berate themselves for not getting better—a Catch-22 if ever there were one. The questions we ask ourselves can be deeply hurtful and harmful. They are more accusatory than inquiring. Take a look at the following list of self-defeating questions. Do you hear these thoughts circling around in your mind, often at a subconscious level? It may help to read the subtext of these questions, which I include in italics.

- What did I do to deserve this? (*I am a victim. Poor me.*)
- Why can't I just grit my teeth and bear this? (*I am weak. I'm a wuss.*)
- Why aren't I doing more? (*I am lazy. I'm a slug.*)
- Why can't I remember anything? (*I am dumb. Maybe I have brain damage.*)
- Why can't I heal myself? (*I am incompetent. I am defective.*)
- Why would anyone want to be with me? (*I am unworthy. I will be alone forever.*)
- Why is everyone disappointed with me? (*Everyone judges me. Why do I keep letting people down?*)
- When can I finally stop hiding my pain from others? (*I can never be myself. They won't love me if they knew the real me.*)
- Why can't I work and contribute to the world? (*I am useless. I am worthless.*)

What if you take these statements and turn them around a bit? "Why" questions are all too often self-blaming and self-defeating. Instead of asking "Why?" perhaps you can begin by asking questions that start with "How?" or "What?" Let's reframe these questions in ways that emphasize motivation, courage, and self-discipline while also acknowledging positive, self-motivating ways of thinking:

- I don't deserve to be in chronic pain—what are the steps I can take to learn how to live with my pain and overcome it? (*I am not a victim; rather, I am a survivor.*)
- How can I use my inner strength, courage, and tenacity to tackle the obstacles in front of me? (*I am powerful. I am competent.*)
- What can I do? What steps can I take? (*I am willing to do whatever it takes.*)
- What can I learn that will be most helpful to me? (*I am smart. I am eager to learn.*)
- How can I use my mind, body, emotions, and spirit to heal myself? (*I am able to find balance in my life.*)
- How can I help my loved ones as they seek to help me? (*I am worthy of their love and attention. Others can help me.*)
- How can I gently remind myself that I am doing the best I can and the people who love me know that, too? (*No one is judging me, especially not as harshly as I am judging myself.*)
- How can I begin to be open and honest about my pain, grief, anger, sadness, and fear—and stop hiding and isolating from others? (*I want—and need—to be myself. It's okay to be vulnerable.*)
- How can I take care of myself and at the same time be of service to others? (*I am useful. Helping others will help me.*)

UNTHINKING THOUGHTS

Thoughts are constructs of your mind composed of electro-chemical reactions among thousands of the billions of nerve cells responsible for relaying messages through trillions of connections (synapses). Each of those trillions of connections transmits about one signal per microsecond, although some specialized synapses relay up to one thousand signals per second—and in ways that are not yet understood, even by neuroscientists, those signals generate thoughts.

All of our thoughts are simply random, floating, fleeting bits of electrical and chemical energy that are—not so simply—the product of myriad neurological reactions taking place in your brain. I like the analogy comparing thoughts to a standing wave in a vast sea of neurons. Picture it in your mind's eye. A wave builds and breaks and disappears, then another wave forms and folds back into the foaming sea, and on it goes, endlessly. Just imagine that your mind is like an ocean, filled with teeming life that is ever diving and surfacing, repeatedly influenced by the "weather" of emotions, events, and experiences, never static, always changing. And deep underneath the teeming sea of your thoughts is a place of calm, quiet, and peace.

Just like waves, your thoughts come and go—and after a while, they *disappear*. They may reappear again and again but once you learn to recognize them, you can diminish their power and credence. As you read the following story, notice how Ashley tackles her negative thoughts about feeling like "a wimp" and not being able to handle life without creating pain. Rather than letting those automatic judgments run away with her (with all their attendant emotions of anger, anxiety, fear, shame, guilt, and so on), she gently tosses out a *but*.

ASHLEY'S STORY

My pain was in the form of headaches. They were chronic, debilitating headaches that would last for days and months with no reprieve. This started in 1998. I had a job that was very stressful—not the job itself, but business politics that ended with my whole team being laid off. I quickly began seeing a neurologist, which was the beginning of being prescribed more medications than one body should ever have. I had my first bout with addiction in 2001, after being prescribed fentanyl. That was short-lived, and I quickly got it under control, or so I thought.

I went to many doctors, tried everything they suggested, took all the medicine they prescribed. I also had several surgeries that were guaranteed to fix the pain. Nothing worked. I finally ended up seeing a neurologist who truly believed in the severity of my pain. This, however, led to an abundance of prescriptions, each one in mass quantities of pills allowed each month. It wasn't just painkillers—I took muscle relaxers, anti-depressants, and sleeping pills. The works. That's when the real problems began, in 2007. I began taking more pills than instructed, mostly so I would sleep. And I slept most of the time, because I was always in pain. I was miserable.

Reluctantly, in April 2011, I checked into LVRC. I was there seven weeks. In that time I learned how the medicines were contributing to my ongoing pain. I learned valuable techniques to live in a world where pain is present, but does not have to be the number one factor of each day. Now, three years later, my headaches are almost completely gone. When I do have a headache, I take Advil. That's it. My life no longer revolves around pain. Any physical discomfort I have is never severe enough to keep me from functioning. I do struggle a little bit with feeling like I'm a wimp. I mean, why can't I just handle my life better without my body creating pain? *But* I remind myself that every person has issues they have to deal with, and this is mine.

Everyone has "issues," Ashley reminds herself, and that awareness is a deep, reassuring comfort, helping her feel less alone. Knowing that her pain was increased by the medications she was taking puts control back in her hands and changes the previous automatic thought, "My head hurts, therefore I need more meds" to "It's not so bad, I can handle it." Today she takes no opioids, anti-anxiety or sleep meds—she doesn't need them! When she has a headache, she might take an over-the-counter pain reliever or just wait to see whether being involved in an activity helps her forget the headache. Pain no longer rules her life.

I will never forget a conversation I had with Ashley one morning in the lunchroom, when she was in treatment. She had the brightest, happiest look on her face.

"What's up?" I said.

"For the first time in over ten years, I don't have a headache today!" she responded with a big smile.

"How do you feel about that?" I asked, matching her smile. I did not expect her answer.

"I feel naked," she said. In that second her smile turned to a frown. "Like something is missing from my life."

Ashley had become so accustomed to living with headaches that she did not feel normal when her headache wasn't there. We spent some time talking that day, as we did many other days during her seven weeks in treatment. She told me the first emotion she felt was excitement . . . then fear . . . then confusion, sadness, embarrassment, and self-doubt.

"I believed that I would have a headache for the rest of my life," Ashley explained. "I thought getting off all my meds was ridiculous. My meds were the only thing making my life and the pain bearable.

So, when I started to see evidence that I might be getting better—holy cow! How exciting! However, on the flip side of that same emotion was fear. Fear that the pain would come back at any minute. Fear that the relief wouldn't last. Fear that I might feel better while at LVRC, but that the pain would come back when I got home.

"And then, and this thought really shocked me—what happens if I get my life back?" Ashley said. "Is this really happening? Is it even possible? And if it is, what do I do now? I've lived the last thirteen years with pain as my identity. More and more I had excused myself from life because I was hurting too badly. I didn't require much (if anything) from myself. Neither did anyone else. If I really am going to feel better, what do I do now? I haven't worked in years. Do I have the discipline required to get back my life and maintain this pain-management type of lifestyle that they're teaching me here?"

I knew it was absolutely critical that we talk about these thoughts and connected emotions because there was a real possibility that Ashley could re-create her headaches just by thinking about them, especially if she was unaware of these inner dialogues. People do that—they start to feel better and then the old patterns of thinking return, and riding right along with the thoughts and the emotions comes the pain.

What we are up against here is called cognitive dissonance, the feeling of uncomfortable tension that comes from holding two conflicting thoughts in your mind at the same time. The dissonance in this case was that Ashley believed something about herself ("I don't deserve to be pain free") and then an experience occurred that called that belief into question ("I am pain free"). Because dissonance is uncomfortable, we sometimes create or re-create a reality that is congruent with our core belief (in Ashley's case, "I will always have headaches").

ARE YOU SAYING THE
PAIN IS ALL IN MY HEAD?

Right about now, as you are reading these paragraphs, you might be getting irritated and annoyed with me. "Are you blaming me for the pain?" you might be thinking. "Are you saying that I created this whole thing, that I'm responsible, that my 'maladaptive' thoughts, as you call them, keep pushing me right back into the pain?"

This is obviously rough territory and it will take some skill for you to navigate through the rocky terrain. It is true that you may become so deeply connected to your pain that it becomes your identity. I've caught myself time and time again thinking about my back pain with a lot of negativity. I'm "attached" to this pain—it grabs me and holds me and shakes me up. I get angry. I swear at my back as if it has its own identity, as if it is somehow separate from me.

But knowing what I know about the way the mind works, right then, right there, I've learned to challenge those thoughts even though they often seem to have sharp teeth. They bite into me and they don't let go until I consciously, carefully work on loosening their hold and letting them release me. And the way I do that, which gets easier and easier with practice, is to remind myself that my thoughts are just constructions of my mind. They just *seem* to sink their canines into me, when in truth they don't have an independent existence outside of me. The thought that they have teeth is merely a . . . *thought.* Just another one of those troublesome, irksome fabrications of my busy, bouncing mind.

And yet even when I have a relatively pain-free day, I often get new toothy thoughts! "Things are going too well," I think. The disturbing thoughts start as a flicker in my subconscious. When I start paying attention—*noticing* the thoughts—they sound something like this: "Sure, I feel pretty good right now, but just wait, it won't last." I hear that a lot from my patients. "Yeah, I feel good today, but it's not going to last, it never lasts. So, I'd better not hope for it or wish for it, because it's too good to be true." It's common for people to fear that the relief of pain won't last. But these fears also tend to disappear if we don't cultivate and inflate them. Try to enjoy the reprieve while you have it and remember that negative thoughts are more like soap bubbles than rabid, vicious animals. One good poke and they're gone—*poof!*—just like that.

I have to stress the importance of *noticing*—paying attention to your thoughts, bringing them from the subconscious to conscious awareness. If you are not aware of the stories being concocted by your mind, they will affect you without your knowledge. So, here's how I might respond when patients express the fear that feeling good or being pain-free will disappear: "Well, if the message is that this day, this hour without pain is too good to be true, then you will sabotage it sooner or later." Or I might say, "Why not enjoy the pain-free time for as long as it lasts? It may last much longer than you think and, of course, it may be gone in a moment."

My patients are not always happy with me when I suggest they take a different perspective on their situation. In fact, some get pretty riled up, automatically assuming that I am accusing them of intentionally causing or prolonging their pain by thinking bad thoughts. Far from it—remember, I know from my work, my training, and my own personal experience that all pain is real. Your thoughts, on the other hand, are not real, and you can challenge negative, harmful thought patterns and begin the process of replacing them—right here, right now—with new ways of thinking about your pain that will loosen its tenacious hold on your mind, body, and spirit.

THE WAY "IN" AND "OUT"

We all have loads of conjured-up negative thoughts—that's just the way it is with our mind, which seems to magnify the negatives and disregard the positives. When you learn to confront unhelpful thoughts and the emotions that cling to them, however, you will discover both a way "in" and a way "out."

Self-knowledge and *awareness* are the way "in." Understanding that negative thoughts generate negative emotions is, in truth, life-changing. Most of us believe that our emotions are created by actual events—someone looks at us "funny" and we feel embarrassed or ashamed. "He made me feel bad" or "You made me angry" are totally false statements. In reality, every experience you have is the product of the electrochemical wizardry of those billions of neurons and trillions of synapses that manufacture thoughts in your brain, which instantaneously create feelings and emotional responses.

In a very real sense, we're dealing with smoke and mirrors. Our thoughts (and the emotions they produce) only seem more and more real and tangible if we grab on to them and commit them to memory by repeating them or ruminating on them. Even then, they are not *real*. The more we reflect on them and act on them, however, the more real they seem and soon we're weaving stories that entangle us in their many threads.

For years Ashley had been told that she needed medications to deal with her headaches. She came to believe that she would always have headaches; they were just a part of her, a part of her nature, her very being. The headaches became so much a part of her story and her identity that when they went away in treatment, she felt "naked" without them. With time, patience, and hard work, Ashley learned how to tell herself a new, headache-free story, one that was more compatible with her new, headache-free life.

The way "out" is to step away from useless and potentially destructive thoughts-beliefs-stories and create a new story. Please understand that I am not simply advocating for "positive thinking." You cannot transcend chronic pain by seeding your mind with positive thoughts that deny the reality of your discomfort, sorrow, and loss. Blocking out or walling off unpleasant or negative thoughts and feelings only leads to self-deception and, in effect, more pain. You hurt and you grieve— that is reality, *your* reality. You mourn for the parts of yourself that you have lost, the life you once had and the future you once imagined for yourself. As my former therapist and now my dear friend Amy always says: "Feel what you feel as long as you need to, and then, when you're ready, move on."

When you are able to acknowledge and accept self-loss, you can move forward. I'll show you how.

CHANGING THE WAY YOU THINK

Let's get right down to it. This table is adapted and expanded from psychiatrist David Burns's "definitions of cognitive distortions" in his groundbreaking book *Feeling Good: The New Mood Therapy*.

12 Ways of Thinking That Get Us into Trouble
(otherwise known as cognitive distortions)

1. **Thinking in black and white:** Your world is divided into good/bad, black/white, perfect/imperfect, with no gray or shaded areas. "*I am always in terrible pain.*" Perfection is the goal and when you fall short (which is inevitable because no one is perfect), you automatically think "failure." "*I can't do anything right.*" "*I am a loser.*"

continues

continued

2. **Making sweeping assumptions:** One slipup and you imagine an ongoing and endless string of defeats. *"Yesterday my pain was a 4 out of 10 but today it's a 5. It's just going to get worse—I bet it will be an 8 by dinnertime. Because I am in pain now, it means I will always be in pain!"*

3. **Focusing on the negative:** All you need is one negative thought or event and all the positive thoughts and emotions disappear. Your perspective narrows (like blinders on a horse) and your vision clouds. *"My glass is always half-empty." "Life is just one misfortune after another. Poor me. They should just shoot me and put me out of my misery."*

4. **Rejecting the positive:** Good things that happen to you are discounted and rejected. Negative thoughts prevail despite the positive experiences that are also part of your life. *"Sure, I had less pain with the breathing exercise, but it didn't last, so it means nothing." "People in group seem to like me . . . they must want something from me."*

5. **Mind reading:** With no facts to support your assumptions, you conclude that someone doesn't like you or is judging you. You have no need to check out the facts because you simply *know* what others are thinking about you (you actually take some pride in your ability to read the minds of other people). *"The nurses are talking about me behind my back and I bet they think I'm faking my pain scores."*

6. **Fortune-telling:** Things are not going to turn out well, you just know it—you feel it in your gut. Like mind reading, fortune-telling is wishful, negative thinking. *"I just know what's going to happen in physical therapy. They will make me exercise, pushing me too hard and too fast, and my pain will get much worse."*

7. **Catastrophizing:** Misery and mayhem lie ahead and every little ache or pain, or every slipup, big or small, is just another sign of upcoming disaster. *"My wife isn't answering the phone, which means she's mad at me and is probably going to divorce me."* Or *"This soreness means I have a new disk herniation and will need surgery that will land me in a wheelchair."*

continues

continued

8. **Minimizing:** Small gains, pain-free moments, good days mean nothing in the big scheme of things and so you shrink them into insignificance. *"Well, I had a good day but it's just one day out of hundreds of bad ones."*

9. **Letting your emotions rule:** Feelings appear to be the reality of your situation. If you feel it, it must be true. *"I am so sad, I wish I was dead."* Or *"I lost my temper again even though I promised that I wouldn't. I'm such a mess!"*

10. **Getting stuck in shoulda, coulda, woulda:** Directed at self, the result of such thinking is guilt and shame; directed at others, the result is irritation, bitterness, resentment, and anger. *"I know I should be able to overcome this pain, I probably could, and I would if I hadn't been in that car accident and the surgeons hadn't botched the operation. I should never have had that operation."*

11. **Labeling:** Negative labels are used in an attempt to simplify an overwhelmingly complex situation and make some kind of sense out of the world. *"I'm a wimp." "I'm weak and pathetic." "My friends are selfish and self-centered." "My children are lazy." "My spouse is an enabler." "My doctor is incompetent."*

12. **Blaming yourself:** You blame yourself for everything negative that happens to you. *"If I were a more upbeat person, my friends would visit more often." "I never should have taken that last ski run when I fractured my ankle." "I should have known better than to take all those drugs, why didn't I see this coming?"*

Now let's take some time to chart how negative, self-critical thought patterns can generate emotions and mood states that directly impact our actions and ability to function.

Thought Pattern Chart

Thought	Emotions	Irrational Response	Reasonable Response
I'm in too much pain to get out of bed and do anything; every time I move, I hurt.	Fear Depression	I'd better stay in bed all day and take a sleeping pill even though it's eleven a.m.	The pain isn't going to kill me and I know movement is good for me—so I'd better get moving!
My friends and family members think I'm pathetic and no longer want to spend time with me.	Self-pity Loneliness Guilt	I'd rather be alone anyway, so I want everyone to just leave me be.	It's not easy to see someone you love in chronic pain, but I know my family and friends love me. They need me as much as I need them.
I've been to dozens of doctors and not one of them treats me with respect. This new doctor doesn't believe that I'm in pain.	Anger Frustration Resentment Blame	I'm not going back to that doctor; she just cares about her paycheck.	I need to meet this doctor one more time to see whether my perceptions are correct. If they are, I will find a doctor who understands my pain and whom I can trust.
I am always going to be in chronic pain.	Anxiety Helplessness Hopelessness Despair	I should just give up and end it now.	I can learn how to live and function with chronic pain and create a good life for myself.

CREATE YOUR
"THOUGHT PATTERN" CHART

Take a blank piece of paper, turn it vertically, and create four columns titled "Thought," "Emotions," "Irrational Response," and "Reasonable Response," as in the chart. Write down your thought patterns as they occur to you. You don't need to create a list from memory; just note your thoughts when they arise. Next, list the emotions that come from these thought patterns. After several days you should have a pretty good list of self-critical thoughts and related emotions, which may or may not mirror some of the thoughts and emotions in this chart.

Now turn your attention to the Irrational and Reasonable Response columns. You can take as long as you like to work on your chart, just keep it close by. You may want to keep a chart on your bedside table—writing down your thoughts and emotions might even help you fall sleep or get back to sleep if you wake up in the middle of the night with disturbing thoughts. Again, feel free to continue to add to this list as new thoughts come to mind. If you're wondering how to tell whether a thought is irrational, write it down, take a breath, and ask yourself: "Is this true or not?" You will always know the answer to that question.

Consider this an ongoing exercise that you can expand as thoughts and emotions arise. You will become more proficient at recognizing and articulating both your reasonable and irrational responses as you continue to add to the list. Feel free to go back and add new interpretations or insights. Keep the list handy and when you are feeling stuck in a self-destructive thinking pattern, revisit the "Reasonable Response" column to help you get free from those bothersome thoughts.

Of course, the key to identifying thoughts, catching and eventually reprogramming them, is to *notice* them *when* they arise. Our thoughts often come and go so fast that we are unaware of their existence, but we can't help but notice the powerful emotions they provoke and we respond to the emotion as if the thought never occurred. By keeping a thought pattern chart, you will learn how to pay closer attention to your thoughts and gain a better understanding of how negative (irrational) thought patterns can negatively affect your day. If you pay close attention, you will clearly see the irrational nature of many of your thoughts. Of course, over time, you will get used to noticing them and then be able to do something about them!

When I have an irrational thought or find myself mind reading ("He must not like me because he sneers at me"), I stop myself before the thought spins out of control. I try to "see" the thought in my mind and correct it, saying to myself, "Oh, he sneers at everyone; it's not personal—in fact, it has nothing to do with me." As for this particular irrational thought, I try to keep in mind what an AA sponsor told me a long time ago: "How they look at you and what they say has less to do with you than with them." Remembering that truth is part of the work of healing, and the payoff is finding comfort rather than distress in your thoughts.

Kathy tells a story about taking her children to the pediatrician where a receptionist was rude to her. Suddenly depressed and out of sorts, Kathy "caught" her negative thoughts ("Why is she so mean? I didn't do anything to her!") and asked one of the nurse practitioners whether the receptionist was having a rough day. "She has an autistic son, and her husband told her this morning that he wants a divorce," the nurse confided.

"That simple interaction was a turning point in my life," Kathy says. "I realized that we are all struggling with one difficulty or another and those problems seep into our relationships. When someone is gruff or unfriendly to me, I tell myself, 'They must be having a bad day.' And I try hard not to add to their unhappiness by taking it personally."

FREE-WRITING

One powerful way to disconnect from your thoughts is through writing. When you write down a thought, you're immediately creating a physical space between you and that thought. That space is then associated with the physical sensations of vision and touch. Somehow your nervous system can internalize that space, helping you detach from your swirling, racing thoughts.

—DAVID HANSCOM, MD, *BACK IN CONTROL*

Years ago Dr. Hanscom suggested that I incorporate free-writing into our treatment program as a technique to help patients unwind the neural circuits involving anxiety, fear, and anger. I am now convinced that free-writing—recording your thoughts in a notebook or legal pad or on a piece of scrap paper, and then throwing away the piece(s) of paper—is one of the most important strategies you can use to distance yourself from negative emotions, including guilt, shame, resentment, apprehension, panic, rage, and self-pity. If negative thoughts create distressing emotions—and of course they do—then putting those thoughts on paper gets them out of your mind, into the light of day, where you can see them and then—best of all—get rid of them.

Many of my patients find an amazing and unexpected release in free-writing. As one patient explained, "Free-writing is what worked for me. They say you use a different part of your brain when you write and you can let go of your thoughts and feelings. In treatment I wasn't sleeping well, and I would get up in the middle of the night and write and write and write about how angry I was. It helped a lot. And it's powerful to tear up what I had written—not reread it—and just toss it in the trash."

Try to keep in mind that free-writing is not intended to make you a better writer or to leave you with information you will use at some future time. Instead, it will enable you to dump unhealthy thoughts onto the page and then discard them, literally. If you do this regularly (at least a few times per week, as I do), it will help you disconnect the circuits of unhealthy negative thinking, thus releasing you from feelings of hopelessness and despair that tend to get stirred up by negative thoughts. And, over time, your pain will decrease.

Here are some suggestions to guide you in your free-writing:

- Put pen or pencil to paper (it's best to write longhand rather than type on a keyboard).
- Write as fast as you can—really, the faster the better!
- Don't pay any attention to penmanship, punctuation, or format.
- Forget about paragraphs, commas, capitals, transitions, or even making sense. Just write spontaneously, letting whatever comes out of your mind (and heart) get deposited on the page.
- Don't stop—keep going until you've written a page or two (feel free to write as much as you want, of course).
- If you get stuck, write about getting stuck!
- *Do not judge* what you write as you write it. Sure, you may take off in some strange or even uncomfortable directions, but that is the

point of the exercise—to just take off, let go, let fly. You may end up somewhere unexpected and eye-opening, even enlightening.

- *Do not read what you have written*—this really is the key to the process.
- Finally, and most important, crumple up the paper and toss it into the wastebasket. Or tear it into pieces. Or shred it. Or, as some people prefer, you can even burn it!

JOURNALING

Journaling is different from free-writing in that you write your thoughts and feelings down with the intent of keeping them and having the option to revisit them. Free-writing is uncensored ("spewing" as one patient put it), whereas journal writing is more often reflective, often guided by the intent of reaching a deeper understanding—and perhaps acceptance—of yourself and your life. In our journals we express our confusion and doubts as well as our joys and triumphs. We begin to see ourselves more clearly through time, as an evolving person, changing, growing, becoming.

When Ellen first came to treatment, her free-writing was almost violent at times. Once, she even shredded the paper after she wrote obscenities about her pain and repeated over and over again, "I hate it I hate it I hate it!!!!!!!!" As time passed, she found herself more comfortable with journaling assignments and developed a regular practice of writing about her thoughts and feelings. She often referred to her journal entries in her counseling sessions, gaining further insights into the process of her long life with pain and her emerging path toward healing.

Think of journaling as an opportunity to look inward, more deeply knowing yourself, your desires, and motivations, and asking the big questions about your life. "Who am I? What do I really want? Why am I here?" are the questions we often ask in our journals. One of the great discoveries you might make is that your deepest "wants" and "needs" are not related to the material world (more money, a bigger house, expensive clothes or shoes, greater prestige) but to the spiritual realities of honesty, respect, trust, faith, hope, and love that give real meaning to your life. When you journal, you record these thoughts and feelings on paper, affirming their significance.

Marie, 60, wrote this journal entry two days after she was admitted to treatment. A second back surgery to correct spinal injuries related to a car accident had failed to relieve her pain, and she came to treatment after overdosing on the high doses of OxyContin and morphine prescribed by her doctor.

Today I met my anger, my anxiety, and decided to breathe into it, wow the anger that came up was so debilitating—it was so hard to take another breath and to actually stay with just one inhale and then concentrate on the out breath. So much stored up emotional baggage—feeling like I have not been heard—feeling that others don't want to hear what I feel. As long as I go along with my husband, everything is smooth—I don't rock the boat—there are no long silences, like I have said something wrong. Trying to share with the one you love who you really are and them just looking at you like they are so uncomfortable so you change the subject to make others happy. You keep giving up your life to make others happy. They become so used to me doing that that they think this is who I am. I try to tell them who I am. I am a spiritual being having a human experience.

Marie kept her journal and continued to write in it for several years. A few months after she left treatment, still struggling with anxiety and anger, she wrote a journal entry addressed to "Voice." When I asked her who or what the word *voice* meant to her, she said: "The voice is *me* going over and over these questions in my head: 'What to do? How am I going to be able to live with this pain? What *is* this pain?'"

Dear Voice:
    Please let me know if it is safe to write down my deepest fears full of fear, hate anxiety selfishness. Am I safe? I am so scared that the stuff inside of me is so full of hate. I hate the word HATE, it's ugly I have always tried to cover up when I am being hateful, vindictive, judging, scared, impatient, ugly thoughts, scared so much fear covering it up so no one will see it covering it up by trying to see the positive in everything, even the pain the pain keeps me on the spiritual path, the hell with that!!! I hurt like hell most of the time it hurts so much to move thru my life thinking there is something

wrong with watching & feeling how others walk thru their life, how do they do it, it's not fair why me? It hurts to get up in the morning and move. I am so angry at GOD for putting me thru this. I am so much better than this kind of life why me "Why me?" It's not fair wanting to be a part of life and having to stop what I am doing and acknowledge this pain is so frustrating. I am so angry at life I look at the insanity and I am devitalized sad angry appalled, sicknessed. I don't want to be a part of this insanity but I am. I don't know how to handle it. Please tell me how to handle what I feel all around me. I don't want to be a part of it, I want to go home. I am searching for connection to you to feel the love, the gratitude the peace inside my soul. The knowing that I have some kind of purpose here. Speaking up I don't have a voice, please help me to find my voice.

Three months later, Marie's writings reflect a significant shift in her perceptions and attitudes:

Loving my self, learning to know that I am loved beyond thoughts. To know I am loved beyond anything I can ever imagine is my truth, it's all there. It is feeling the creator's love at all times in this life. It is accepting that I am loved beyond anything I can ever imagine. It is seeing, feeling the beauty that is always everywhere. If I knew at every moment of my life that I am loved I would fall at my feet.

And, a few weeks later:

Thank you for my arms & hands & fingers
Thank you for my amazing sense of taste
Thank you for my wonderful sense of smell
Thank you for my precious sense of touch
Thank you for my eyes that enable me to see everything
Thank you for my beautiful mind & brain.
Thank you cells, thank you organs for working perfectly.
Thank you for my strong and healthy heart!

In one of her most recent journal entries, the only entry with a title, Marie wrote:

The Magic

I am grateful for my husband.
I am grateful for hot water.
I am truly grateful for heat.
I am grateful for that first sip of coffee in the morning.
I am grateful for the word grateful and how when writing it,
    it just flows.
I am grateful for my health, to be able to walk, bicycle.
I am grateful for my bed.
I am grateful for my home.
I am grateful for cleaning supplies.
I am grateful for my washing machine, I am grateful
    for my dryer.
I am grateful for my car.
I am grateful for my food, juicing.
I am grateful for my health.

These remarkable journal entries illustrate the progress Marie has made in addressing her unhealthy thought patterns, finding the positive realities in her life, searching for meaning, and moving steadily toward recovery. Today, she rates her pain as 1 or 2 out of 10, although she still has flare-ups that may last for an hour or, sometimes, even for a day or two. At those times she writes in her journal, chronicling her thought and feelings, and reading back through her past entries to remind herself to accept the pain when it comes, knowing it won't last forever.

COGNITIVE BEHAVIORAL THERAPY

The tables and techniques I've suggested in the last several pages are congruent with a school of psychotherapy called rational emotive behavior therapy (REBT) and cognitive behavioral therapy (CBT). Today, *cognitive behavioral therapy* is an umbrella term used for various therapies that focus on faulty thinking that causes distortions in the way we see and react to others and our world, leading to disorders in our emotions and behavior.

In his fascinating book *Feeling Good*, David Burns, MD, explains that CBT is based on three simple principles that I expand upon here:

PRINCIPLE 1: Your thoughts and cognitions actually create— manufacture!—your moods and emotions. A cognition is more than a thought because it includes your belief system, attitudes, interpretations, and perceptions of the world. What you are thinking about right now is responsible for whatever mood you might be in.

Suppose you are thinking about a recent tornado that killed dozens of people. You might be asking yourself why you deserve to complain about your own pain when there is so much misery in the world, when death and destruction can come ferociously and unexpectedly out of what was only recently a clear blue sky. After all, you're alive, even if your pain is pretty awful. "This is my life," you think, "constant, unrelenting pain."

You think back to the tornado victims and immediately you ask yourself, "Why am I so selfish and self-centered?" That question stings! "Why is it always about me?" you wonder, suddenly feeling blue and slightly guilty. Your heart goes out to all those people whose houses and lives have been destroyed. "Life sucks," you think. "What's the meaning of it all, anyway?" By now, you're really down in the dumps. You pull the covers over your head, shut your eyes, and try to escape through sleep and a few pills.

The very moment that a thought comes into your head—with or without you realizing it—if you latch on to it by judging it, ruminating on it, or getting hooked by it, you will have an emotional response. That's CBT Principle #1.

PRINCIPLE 2: When you are feeling anxious, fearful, frustrated, angry, guilty, depressed, or any of the other myriad emotions that come with the territory of chronic pain, your thoughts can get dark and threatening. "Your thoughts are dominated by a pervasive negativity," explains Dr. Burns. "You perceive not only yourself but the entire world in dark, gloomy terms. What is even worse—you'll come to believe things *really are* as bad as you imagine them to be . . . this bleak vision creates a sense of hopelessness." The storm clouds are building as your negative thoughts generate damaging emotions that in turn create destructive belief systems built on a swelling sense of despair.

PRINCIPLE 3: The whole construct of thoughts, emotions, and belief systems represent a distorted or maladaptive reality. What you think you know to be true—what you believe is reality, what you feel in your bones are honest-to-goodness, genuine, valid emotions—may be, and often is an illusion. Dr. Burns calls this "mental slippage," which brings to mind the images in the Joni Mitchell song "Both Sides Now," where she compares clouds to castles and canyons. Our thoughts are like those clouds—illusive, deceptive, captivating constructs of our imagination. It is their captivating nature (read: captive) that drags in emotions as a fishnet traps swimming creatures, and these strong emotions ensure that the thoughts will snag in the very cells of our body (cellular memory). All too often it's the "illusions" we recall.

ACCEPTANCE

Accepting the fact that your thoughts ignite your emotions, which, in turn, create destructive, reality-distorting belief patterns, is an essential starting point for change. Furthermore, accepting the fact that you have chronic pain and thus it will be with you for a long time—maybe for your whole lifetime—offers a realistic approach that puts you in a position to move forward and begin to make the changes that will allow you to live—and thrive—*with* your pain.

I am asking you to pay attention to your pain rather than cover it up with such statements as "No one wants to hear about my problems," "I need to be strong and stop complaining," "Keep a stiff upper lip," or "A lot of people have bigger problems than mine." I'm asking you to *lean into your pain*, regardless of how unpleasant it may be. I'm asking you to be interested in the experience you are having—even curious about its dimensions and characteristics.

Right about now you might be thinking: "But I don't want this pain. What do you mean, lean in, I want to lean *out*! I just want to get away from this pain, I want to get rid of it, be done with it!" Or, at the opposite extreme, your thoughts might serve to isolate you even further: "Just leave me alone with my pain." "Nobody understands what it is like to be in constant pain—after all, how could they?"

To which I might respond: "What I hear you saying is that you are so committed to your pain—or to the hope that you can eliminate it completely—that your whole life is about pain. Pain has become most of what you think about, your identity." I pause before I ask, "Are you so committed to your pain that you are willing to accept a second-class life?"

Life can get better. I have yet to meet a person in chronic pain who doesn't desperately want to believe that statement. Can you genuinely get in touch with the part of you that thinks and feels in this way: "I want a better life than I've had up until now. I don't want to be ruled by my pain. I don't want a second-class life!"

If I assure you that your life can get better, then the question becomes: What can you do to start the process? In addition to CBT, two therapeutic approaches that can be very useful at this point are dialectical behavioral therapy (DBT) and acceptance and commitment therapy (ACT), both outgrowths of cognitive behavioral therapy.

DIALECTICAL BEHAVIORAL THERAPY

DBT is a therapeutic process that deals with almost every type of emotional issue, focusing on the individual's social skills and interactions with the goal of developing a sense of self and alleviating the empty, hopeless feelings so many people have. Mindfulness is a key component of DBT (see Chapter 7 for an in-depth discussion of mindfulness), along with skills related to distress tolerance, emotional regulation, and interpersonal effectiveness.

I asked my colleague Elaina Jensen, a psychiatric-mental health and certified addiction nurse practitioner, to offer her perspective on DBT's effectiveness with chronic pain patients.

DBT is very useful for people with chronic pain because it was created for people who are highly sensitive to intense emotion (pain). I will never forget when I learned that the experience of chronic pain is driven in large part by emotions. It's hard enough to deal with an out-of-balance emotional system, but patients with chronic pain come in with both the physical and emotional aspects of pain so, really, they are dealing with close to 100 percent of their system out of balance. And it's likely that these patients have been consistently invalidated regarding the *real* pain they feel.

DBT validates such intense emotions and pain with a technique called radical acceptance, an emotional regulation skill. Creating a validating environment is necessary to empower the clients to take a more active part in their treatment and recovery, beyond pain pills and medications, so they can start to let go of the pain. They learn to connect and validate the pain and then move beyond it through various mindful meditations and techniques. DBT teaches a middle-ground stance by striving to synthesize a balance of acceptance and change, which can be challenging when a person's system of functioning has been centered around pain or the avoidance of pain by taking pain pills.

ACCEPTANCE AND COMMITMENT THERAPY

ACT is geared toward goal-setting and goal-attainment. Unlike CBT, which teaches you to better control your thoughts, feelings, and sensations, ACT focuses on noticing, accepting, and embracing unwanted events. At the heart of ACT is psychological flexibility, which can be understood as the ability to adapt to new circumstances or experiences. Several important steps are involved in this ability to adjust to the ups and downs of life:

1. Focusing attention on problematic thought patterns and neutralizing their negative impact on our emotions (called cognitive defusion)
2. Acceptance, which involves accepting not only your experiences of pain but the constellation of emotions surrounding your pain
3. Identifying your values (what is most important to you in your life)
4. Setting realistic goals that are based on your values
5. Moving forward with a sense of purpose and commitment

Focused attention, acceptance, value identification, realistic goals, and mindfulness will be among your most loyal allies in managing your pain. Let's turn our attention for a moment to the importance of values and identifying what is most meaningful to you as a unique individual.

Finding Meaning in Life

Focusing on values will have a profound impact on both your ability to accept your pain and your motivation to take necessary actions to move beyond a life that is wholly defined by pain. Often in my interactions with my patients I will ask them what is important for them to accomplish in their life, and then just listen as they talk about what means the most to them.

I listen, and I ask questions. The questions I ask—and the questions I encourage you to ask yourself, gently and nonjudgmentally—run along the following lines. (I encourage you to write about them in your journal—each of the questions below can be used as a "topic" for a journal writing exercise.)

- If you didn't have this pain, how would your life be different?
- What do you want your life to stand for?
- How do you resist change in your life?
- Why do you resist change?
- What is the worst thing that would happen if you let your feelings out?
- How can you keep yourself from being overwhelmed?
- Can you envision three goals that would bring joy—and meaning—back into your life?
- What is your pain teaching you about your life?
- What do your symptoms want from you?
- What questions is your pain asking you?
- Where do you feel stuck physically, mentally, emotionally, spiritually?
- What can you do to restore faith in your body's self-healing capabilities and have confidence in your future?
- Why are you experiencing difficulty communicating your thoughts and feelings to others?
- Why do you hide from others—what are you afraid of? What will happen to you if you express your true thoughts and feelings?
- What past losses are you grieving over?
- What will it take for you to let go of your grief?

- How can you bring more balance into your life and respond, rather than simply react, to situations that arise?
- What can you control in your life? What can't you control?

I want to emphasize that my hope is that you always focus on what is meaningful to you. For learning how to live with chronic pain is, at its most basic level, a search for meaning. All human beings are intrinsically motivated to make some kind of sense of their lives, their human experience. If you can't make sense of your pain . . . if you can't find a way to live a quality life with the pain . . . if you can't emerge from your cocoon and become part of a caring community that will bear with you as you struggle to find your way in and through the pain—then I am afraid that the only pathway open to you may be lined with hopelessness and despair.

You do not need to choose that dark, desolate pathway. I hope these "values questions" help you see, acknowledge, and appreciate the multitude of options that are spread out before you.

EXPECTATIONS

Are you willing to believe that good things will happen if you make the commitment to engage in the steps outlined in this and the remaining chapters? Because, really, it all begins right here. If you relentlessly hold on to the belief that you are doomed to live with this level of pain for the rest of your life, then your expectations will most likely continue to come true. If, on the other hand, you believe that trying even just one or two of the techniques and strategies offered in these pages might help you live a fuller, richer life—if what I've said so far rings true for you—then chances are very good that you will improve and have a better life. As with most changes, the more you invest, the greater the gains.

As you read through the following chart, consider how both optimistic and pessimistic expectations can skew reality—and how realistic expectations can help you arrive at a place of balance. Notice the flexible, thoroughly reasonable perspective outlined in column 3. Optimism is great, but we often burden our hopes and expectations of success with specific wishes or goals, and it is this attachment to explicit, identifiable results that causes problems for us ("I'll only be okay if the pain is totally gone." "I expect to be pain free by my fortieth birthday." "I believe I can handle this pain on my own without any outside help"). On the other hand, believing that "I'm at the mercy of fate," or "The pain is only going to get worse as I get older," may create a fatalistic acceptance of ever-worsening pain that destroys confidence in your body's innate healing mechanisms.

Between high hopes and fatalism is a place of honest assessment and determined commitment. Try to find that point of balance in your life by using the powers of your mind to challenge unfounded assumptions and achieve realistic expectations.

Optimistic Expectations	Pessimistic Expectations	Realistic Expectations
I see the cup as half-full.	I see the cup as half-empty.	I see the cup as containing enough water to satisfy my thirst. And there's more where that came from.
I believe that I have total control over my pain level and can manage my pain.	I believe that I will never be able to control my pain level.	There are some things I can do to reduce my pain and live more comfortably.
Pain will not interfere with my life.	Pain has a mind of its own, and I can't do anything about how it affects my life.	Pain may always be part of my life, and I can find ways to live well and coexist with it.
I have faith that the strategies in this book will work to significantly reduce my pain.	I don't have a lot of hope that I can manage my pain on my own, especially without drugs.	I believe that if I am disciplined about putting these strategies into practice, my pain will be manageable and my life will get better.

THE PLACEBO EFFECT

The power of the mind is extraordinary! Hundreds of research studies show that if people in pain believe a placebo (usually a sugar pill or other inert substance) is actually a pain-relieving medicine, more than 25 percent report a substantial decrease in their pain after taking the "medicine." While this may be hard to believe, let me quote Dr. Steven Novella, assistant professor of neurology at Yale University's School of Medicine. Well known for his skeptical approach to alternative medicine techniques, Dr. Novella leaves little doubt in this post on the Science-Based Medicine website that the placebo effect works for people who are experiencing both acute and chronic pain.

> Pain is uniquely amenable to manipulation through mood and expectation . . . studies show that the brain is hardwired to modulate pain based upon expectation . . . putting a positive spin on the potential of a pain intervention is therapeutic.

While it may seem that our expectations are based solely on our internal belief system—what we think will occur, what we want to occur, and what we believe should occur (as well as expectations that lurk beneath our consciousness)—something else is also at work here. At Harvard University, associate professor of medicine Ted Kaptchuk and his research team have been studying placebo effects to find out *how* they work. With the aid of new imaging technologies, such as functional magnetic resonance imaging (fMRI) and positron emission tomography (PET) scans, Kaptchuk's research shows that placebo treatments have a powerful effect on the same areas of the brain that regulate pain perception. In other words, placebos stimulate electrical and chemical responses in the brain that use the same pathways as such drugs as marijuana, hydrocodone, oxycodone, morphine, and heroin, altering electrical and metabolic activity throughout the brain's neurocircuitry to stimulate sensations of pleasure and reward.

I believe the most exciting aspect of this research is the critical importance placed on the doctor-patient relationship and "the ritual" of medicine. "Doctors give subtle cues to their patients that neither may be aware of. They are a key ingredient in the ritual of medicine," Kaptchuk explains in a 2014 *Harvard Magazine* article titled "The Placebo Phenomenon." What kind of "subtle cues" is he talking about? In a study with irritable bowel syndrome (IBS) patients, Kaptchuk and other researchers discovered that the patients who received the most attention from their doctors (at least twenty minutes of listening, thoughtful silences, such reassurances as "I know how difficult this is for you," and compassionate physical contact by touching the patient's hands or shoulders) experienced the greatest relief from the placebo treatments.

This is vital information for you as a patient and for me as a doctor. The way you are treated by your doctor—with coldness or with kindness—will have a profound effect on your experience of pain and the relief you experience from the treatment strategies your doctor utilizes and prescribes. If your doctor is brusque, tight-lipped, arrogant, overbearing, and too busy to pay attention to you, I strongly urge you to search for a different health-care practitioner. Find a doctor who exhibits warmth and compassion, who listens carefully and well, and who doesn't jump to conclusions but thoughtfully considers your words and your emotions. Your thoughts, emotions, and basic well-being are deeply, powerfully affected by the attitudes and empathy of those who are accompanying you on this healing journey. We would all do well to heed the Dalai Lama's words about "real care of the sick":

> When people are overwhelmed by illness, we must give them physical relief, but it is equally important to encourage the spirit through the constant show of love and compassion. It is shameful how often we fail to see that what people desperately require is human affection. Deprived of human warmth and a sense of value, other forms of treatment prove less effective. Real care of the sick does not begin with costly procedures, but with the simple gifts of affection, love and concern.

SIX

RESTORING PHYSICAL BALANCE
Creating a Safe Pathway Between Extremes

Your hand opens and closes, opens and closes.
If it were always a fist or always stretched open,
you would be paralyzed. Your deepest presence
is in every small contracting and expanding,
the two as beautifully balanced and
coordinated as birds' wings.

—RUMI

Try this: Close your hand as tightly as you possibly can. See the skin stretching tight over your knuckles, the veins flattening and stretching, tendons taut. Hold your breath. Are your fingernails digging into your palms? Are you clenching your jaw? Do you feel radiating tension in your shoulders, your back, your neck, head, feet?

Now open your hand. Take a nice deep breath, spread your fingers wide, stretch them to the sky, then exhale, relaxing a little, letting your fingers curl slightly, and resting your hands on your thighs or your lap. How does that feel? Better? Certainly you notice the difference. Your blood is flowing, energy is circulating. Relaxed now, take another deep, breath. Fill your lungs with oxygen and exhale slowly, allowing any residual tension to dissipate as the air leaves your body.

Just as a bird's wings stretch but do not strain, fold but do not stiffen, so can you, through "every small contracting and expanding," learn to fly again. Use Rumi's words as a reminder of the need for balance and coordination, for every opening necessarily involves a closing, every tension includes a release, every inhalation is followed by an exhalation. Sixth-century BC philosopher Lao-tzu described the process of folding and unfolding in this way in his classic Chinese text the *Tao Te Ching*, which has been translated into Western languages more than 250 times:

> *If you want to become whole,*
> *first let yourself become broken.*
> *If you want to become straight,*
> *first let yourself become twisted.*
> *If you want to become full,*
> *first let yourself become empty.*
> *If you want to become new,*
> *first let yourself become old.*

Broken, twisted, empty, old. Is this not how we often feel as people living with chronic pain? I know I sure do, some days. But there is another side to that rather gloomy perspective, for we can become *whole, straight, full, new.* How? Several translations of Lao-tzu end the above stanza with this phrase, the ultimate paradox:

> *If you want to be given everything,*
> *give everything up.*

Surrendering to this truth begins with the mind, as discussed in Chapter 5, but it does not end there. Understanding how your thoughts impact your emotions is only the beginning of the journey to discover a sense of balance in your life. Now we turn to the physical realm—the body and its specific needs. Always remember, though, that any distinction between mind and body is artificial—for mind and body are intimately and intricately connected. In other words, your mind, which is housed in your brain, is part of your body. (Big *duh,* I know, but I stress this because we so often separate mind from body, reasoning—with our mind, of course!—that if an ache or pain is not physical—visible or obvious—it's somehow not legitimate or real.)

FINDING THE MIDDLE PATH

If you are like most people living with chronic pain, you live in a world of excesses or extremes. Perhaps you take handfuls of drugs to ease your pain or you refuse to take any drugs at all. You eat too much or you go on a strict diet. You exercise not at all or you dive headlong into strenuous physical training or extreme sports. You keep to yourself or you immerse yourself in trying to help others, often to the point of neglecting your own needs. You don't get enough sleep or you sleep half the day away. You refuse to try any alternative therapies or you try them all, moving from yoga to acupuncture, meditation, hypnotherapy, Chi Kung, and Reiki, with no clear plan for assessing each method's therapeutic benefits.

Where is the "middle path" between extremes and why is it important for people living with chronic pain to find a balance between extremes? Rumi's luminous words in the opening quotation offer a partial answer to these questions in the image of finding a balance between opening and closing, contracting and expanding, "beautifully balanced and coordinated as birds' wings." Chronic pain has thrown you off balance. The key to regaining balance is to re-create, slowly and gently, that sense of stability and steadiness that will allow you to move forward—to rediscover your wings. I will show you how to do just that.

EXERCISE

Coping with chronic pain depends on a patient's
willingness to exercise and increase productive activity
despite the feeling of pain. Chronic pain management
succeeds when the patient accepts the possibility
of living a useful life in the presence of pain.

—DR. PAUL BRAND

The unmovement syndrome (also called the fear-avoidance syndrome, or kinesiophobia) so common in chronic pain patients *must* be replaced with regular exercise. Physical activity is critically important—even though it may feel bad when you move, the less you move, the more pain you will have. And, just because it *hurts* to move doesn't mean it is causing *harm*.

I exercised my calves and thighs Friday, and today, Sunday, it hurts to walk and even to sit down. But that doesn't mean I've harmed anything—in fact, I know I haven't. It hurts "good" and I know I will ultimately benefit from the workout. "Hurting good" is a theme in this chapter, and I will discuss ways to get you moving again to help you improve your physical condition.

If pain settles in and takes over, you are stuck in unmovement. Here's how a patient explained it: "It hurts when I move so I don't move and the more I don't move, the more it hurts when I move. I'm scared to go to physical therapy, do yoga, even take a walk because any type of activity increases my pain. If I could just lie in bed all day, I wouldn't have any pain."

But here's what I have to say: *"Move anyway, even if it hurts!"* One way to get moving is to ask yourself whether you really want to spend most of the hours of your day lying in bed or in a recliner. You might immediately respond, "Yes, sure, because then I don't have pain." But then ask yourself: "What kind of a life is that? Is this the life I really want?" Remember, I am urging you to find meaning in your life, and movement is part of it. Besides, you *have* to move—you have to go to the bathroom, for example. So, you can begin there. When you go to the bathroom, take a leisurely walk around your house or apartment. After all, you're already up. Spend a few minutes looking out the window. Take several deep breaths, feeling your chest move out, then in as you exhale, contracting and expanding. Gently, slowly, turn your neck to the right and then to the left.

Even those little movements might cause an increase in pain—and, again I say, *"Do them anyway!"* When you move, no matter how small that movement might be at the beginning, you break up pain's power and break down its control over your life. Moving may *hurt* but it will not *harm* unless you overdo it. For that reason, I counsel patients who haven't moved or exercised much or often to consult with a physical therapist or trainer before starting an exercise regime in order to avoid injury. I often hear my patients groaning in their sessions with LVRC's trainer, Jason, but invariably, and with a certain amount of pride, they tell me later that it "hurts good."

Think of finding your "edge"—the boundary between "Ouch, that hurts," and "Oh-my-god, I can't bear it!" Allow yourself to move to the point where it hurts and then go a little bit beyond that point. Push to your limit, always within reason, and then pull back. Then push again, perhaps a little farther this time. Your body will tell you when you reach your "edge," and the more you push to your limit, the more you will discover that activity that was once unbearable is now bearable. Listen carefully and pay close attention, then respond with gentleness and always remember the central thesis of this book—all pain is real. Pay attention to your pain but do not allow it to control your life. You hold the controls—make your pain just a passenger, not the driving force in your life.

These exercises are about finding your edge—and seeing that you can always go further. If you progress by small increments, even micromovements with an eye toward progress, over time you will notice substantial improvement in your ability to move past your "edge" and "hurt good."

"Hurting Good" Guidelines

Hurting good can be bad for you only if you push yourself too far. But how do you know how far to push yourself? How can you find your "edge"? Here are four concrete tips:

1. Stand on your tiptoes for as long as you can—see how long you can last before letting your feet return to the floor. Aim for a few more seconds each time you do this.
2. Lift your arms up toward the ceiling—how far can you go?—try walking your fingers up the wall and make a pencil mark. Each time you do this, go a little higher than the previous time.
3. Tighten the muscles of your abdomen. Hold as long as you possibly can and then relax. Check the time. Next time, do it for a few seconds longer and so on.
4. Twist your neck to one side until it hurts—see where your eyes fall and what you see when you twist. Relax and next time, aim to pass by the mark you got to the time before and so on.

EXERCISES TO COMBAT
THE UNMOVEMENT SYNDROME

The following exercises and practices will lessen your pain over time, even though they almost certainly will cause some initial increase in discomfort. Hang in there. Body parts that are not moved or used for any length of time (back, abdomen, knees, shoulders, necks, hips, etc.) eventually become stiff and essentially frozen. When your movements are restricted, your circulation gets sluggish, and blood oxygen levels drop. Sustained pressure on various parts of your body from lying or sitting too long, poor posture, and general lack of movement all increase muscle tension and can lead to low oxygen levels in the soft tissues of your body, which causes scar tissue to form. Scar tissue is not as flexible and elastic as a healthy muscle, nor does it lengthen and respond like normal muscle. Because scar tissue is weaker and less flexible than normal tissue, it is more prone to injury and more sensitive to pain. Nerves become trapped in the scar tissue, resulting in more pain and dysfunction as well as tingling, numbness, and weakness. As scar tissue builds up, you will experience more limited range of motion, decreased circulation, reduced energy, and more pain.

The good news is that scar tissue does not have to be permanent. Physical therapy, yoga, Chi Kung, massage, and weight bearing, flexibility, and strengthening exercises will help "remodel" scar tissue, loosening adhesions (which feel like knots) and allowing the muscle fibers and connective tissue to realign and return to normal. As the scar tissue is loosened and stretched, you can achieve improved range of motion, restoring normal blood flow and oxygenation—and a noticeable, even remarkable decrease in your pain.

Furthermore, because physical exercise also bumps up the endorphins (your body's natural pain-relieving neurotransmitters), inactivity and immobility often lead to depression and anxiety, which, in turn, feed into the cycle of immobility and intensified pain. For many people the end result is complete loss of function, which, I would argue, is an agonizingly slow way of letting your life force drain away, taking all the joy and wonder of existence along with it.

Moving hurts and, of course, you fear doing anything that will aggravate your pain. So, while it seems to make sense that you should move as little as possible so as to avoid pain, nothing could be more detrimental to your health than unmovement. By stretching and mobilizing joints and other areas of the body, circulation increases, motion improves, and you feel better. Walking, aerobic activities, yoga, stretching, weight bearing, and other forms of exercise will reduce your experience of pain in the following ways:

- Help you maintain a healthy weight, which lessens the stress on your joints, easing that aching feeling deep in your bones
- Increase flexibility, thereby reducing stress and strain on joints and the spine
- Break down the scar tissue that has formed from inactivity
- Loosen up tight muscles, tendons, and ligaments, resulting in increased range of motion and improved function
- Strengthen muscles, thereby taking the load off your joints and bones
- Improve circulation so the bloodstream can carry essential nutrients to tissues and remove toxins that contribute to inflammation and disease
- Enhance mental alertness, long-term memory, attention, and problem-solving abilities. (Our brain, which composes 2 percent of our weight but consumes 20 percent of our energy during the day, needs lots of oxygen-soaked blood.)
- Regulate neurotransmitters (including dopamine, serotonin, norepinephrine, and endorphins) that improve mood and strengthen the neurological messaging systems that your body uses to fight chronic pain

In addition to reducing your pain, research shows that regular exercise will:

- Cut your lifetime risk of general dementia in half
- Reduce the risk of Alzheimer's by 60 percent
- Decrease the risk of more than a dozen types of cancer
- Reduce your risk of heart attack and stroke by improving cardiovascular fitness

What type of exercise will deliver the greatest benefits? Just a little movement makes a big difference—in fact, research shows that even couch potatoes who squirm, wriggle, or fidget show increased benefits over their immobile couch potato friends! I'm not advocating being a squirming, fidgeting couch potato, but there's no denying that even small movements repeated regularly during the day will make a difference—and starting with small movements is fine. The more you move, the more you will want to move, especially if you can tuck away in your memory the fact that any short-term pain involved won't hurt you but will actually reduce your pain in the long run. I love to watch patients walking our outdoor circuit, when just a few weeks earlier they were spending twenty hours of the day in bed. Often they will pair up or walk in groups, and I feel as if I can almost see the healing take place in the way they talk, listen, smile, and laugh together.

What is the ultimate goal you are working toward? Many fitness experts set the "gold standard" as aerobic (heart-pumping) exercise for thirty minutes, two to three times a week. This may seem like a difficult if not impossible objective, but dedication and commitment will help you reach it in time. Patience is key—if it takes you six months or a year to reach your goals, that's just fine. You are the only person who can measure your progress with any accuracy. You are the one who is receiving the benefits of exercise and who can assess the impact of your efforts on the quality of your life.

But where should you start? The following exercises will help you break through your fear of pain. Studies have shown that when your fear diminishes, your pain will as well, and you will regain mobility and confidence. The antidote for the fear-avoidance cycle—a syndrome that affects virtually every person who lives with chronic pain—is slow, gentle exposure to activities with gradual increases in your level of activity as time goes on. As I mentioned, it is likely that you will experience some initial discomfort as you loosen up tight muscles and break down fibrous scar tissue that has built up as a result of inactivity.

Please try to keep these two general guidelines in mind as you read through this section on exercise: (1) Push yourself within reason, always remembering to be gentle with yourself (keep in mind the "Hurting Good Guidelines" on page 139); and (2) Vary your exercise. Constant, repetitive movements put a strain on your body, so alternating different forms of exercise—walking one day, taking a yoga class the next, and doing light aerobic exercise the following day is a sample routine that will prove beneficial (it will also keep you from getting bored with just one type of exercise!).

Walking

Okay, right now, put this book down, get up and go for a walk. Ten steps, fifty steps, or one hundred steps . . . a walk around the block or up and down the stairs . . . a five- or ten-minute stroll if you can manage it. Go slowly at first . . . but go. Do what you can and then push yourself to do just a little bit more each time you go for a walk. I don't want you to be limited by your self-imposed restrictions, but I do want you to be aware of healthy limits. Pace yourself. Notice where it hurts. Remind yourself that you can do it—you don't need to be defined by your pain. But, again, keeping your "edge" in mind is always important. If you are going for a walk, as I reminded a patient recently, go half as far as you think you can, so you can be sure you have enough energy to get back!

Just getting up from your bed or chair will increase your circulation, stretch your muscles, decrease spasms, lubricate your joints, and begin the process of strengthening your muscles and bones. Every day try to push a little harder or go a little bit farther—perhaps from a walk to the kitchen to a stroll around the entire house or from walking up and down one flight of stairs to walking up and down two flights of stairs. Give yourself credit, setting realistic goals and sticking with them. Jot down your accomplishments on a note pad or in your journal. Be pleased with yourself and whatever you accomplish!

Light Aerobic Exercise

The following light to moderate aerobic exercises will help your heart beat faster, which increases your breathing rate, which allows you to take in more oxygen, which helps your cells perform their given tasks (making repairs, cleaning the blood, digesting food, dividing into new cells), which lifts your spirits and generally makes your life better.

Here are some sample aerobic exercises:

- Short walks at a brisk pace—enough to make you feel a little winded but still able to carry on a conversation
- Longer walks (1 or 2 miles) on relatively flat ground
- Leisurely bike rides on flat roads or trails
- Lap swimming (start with one lap or two)
- Water aerobics

- Aerobic dance (Jazzercise, Zumba, Nia, hip-hop, salsa, belly dancing—but remember to take it easy)
- Gentle workouts on exercise machines (rowing or elliptical machines, treadmills, stationary bikes with or without a backrest). Find one or two workouts that suit you and try to alternate.
- Golf (which, as Mark Twain reminds us is really "a good walk spoiled"!)
- Everyday activities, such as mowing the lawn, vacuuming, sweeping, raking, walking up and down the stairs, and, yes, sex

Yoga

Yoga means union—the union of body with consciousness and consciousness with the soul. If you have never done yoga, be sure to find a certified instructor and attend some classes to learn the proper techniques. Many YMCAs and YWCAs offer yoga classes that are often free for members. More and more community centers are also offering classes with reasonable rates. Private studios offer a variety of classes ranging from restorative yoga and gentle yoga to advanced yoga techniques. Talk to the instructor before class to let him or her know about your limitations. Gentle yoga is best for people with chronic pain, but just because the class is called "gentle" doesn't mean you can or should try all the positions.

Always, always go at your own pace. If you feel as though the class exceeds that pace, talk again to the instructor about your challenges and difficulties or find another class. Softness and gentleness must rule the day although, once again, gradually finding your "edge" is also part of yoga practice. Your yoga teacher will most likely ask you to focus on your painful areas, and for many people, this is a little disconcerting as you may have been told—or you've told yourself—it's best to take your mind off the pain, to stop obsessing, and to distract yourself from thinking about the hurting places. But as discussed in Chapter 5, when you stop trying to avoid pain and instead put your attention on what hurts, you often find that the experience of pain shifts and changes. Yogic philosophy interprets this shifting of pain from one area to another as a sign that the pain you feel is due in large part to your perception of pain, rather than the actual pain itself.

I highly recommend *Yoga for Pain Relief* by Kelly McGonigal and *Yoga for Emotional Balance*, by Bo Forbes.

Kathy and I asked two of our favorite yoga teachers, Cheryl Slader in Las Vegas and Robin Hamilton in Walla Walla, to share their thoughts about the benefits of yoga for people living with chronic pain.

Cheryl says:

Yoga connects body, mind, and spirit. It focuses greatly on the life force, prana, breath. It helps you get out of your own way, to come into the present moment and break the cycle of pain and/or addiction that is controlled by your mind. It helps you take the "seat of the witness," watching your thoughts but not attaching to them, realizing that you are not your thoughts, eventually making more space in between the thoughts.

Generally, it takes two to three sessions for most people to "warm up" to yoga. Men like yoga as much as women; in fact, in many classes I have more men than women. Older people may be a bit more reluctant to start yoga but once they try it, they love it. I always counsel people to just do what they can. Even if you just sit in a chair and work on keeping your back straight and breathing deep, you are "doing" yoga. Yoga is a lifestyle, a constant practice, living your life and constantly being observant and curious of the new "now" moment that you find yourself in. Yoga is keeping words like *peace*, *love*, *trust*, and *faith* in your heart always and treating yourself and others kindly.

Robin says:

The practice of yoga is especially helpful for people with chronic pain, primarily because of its focus on the breath. When you are in constant pain, you may withdraw, physically, mentally and emotionally. By becoming more in tune with your breath, as a yoga practitioner, you can access the greatest friend you'll ever know. Depending on the breath practice—and there are many—the mind can be sharpened or stilled, the body can be awakened or calmed. If you suffer from chronic pain, learning these simple techniques may help you find a way to relieve your pain, much like breath practices used in childbirth.

You can also become mindful of your internal dialogue, often changing a negative conversation with yourself to a positive one. The result can be profound.

Practicing yoga poses will help you open your body over time. By slowly learning balancing poses, deep binds, twists, and by linking postures with breath, you'll have the opportunity to acknowledge and deal with emotions that may arise when something is difficult. You will also learn, by practicing compassion with yourself, to deal with physical limitations. With consistent practice, your body will change for the better.

The point of yoga is to experience peace on the mat, and to take it out into the world. It is an empowering and life-affirming practice that can be a comfort and a balm to anyone suffering with chronic pain.

Most important of all—yoga is fun! And fun helps relieve pain.

▪ ▪ ▪

Note: I'd also like to emphasize the benefits of restorative yoga for people with chronic pain. Practiced with a trained instructor, restorative yoga is a gentle, soothing method, utilizing props (bolsters, blankets, balls, blocks, towels, eye pillows, cushions, chairs, and walls) to fully support the body. Poses are typically held for longer periods than in other types of yoga practice, sometimes as long as twenty, or even thirty minutes. These soothing, well-supported poses eliminate unnecessary straining and very gently loosen stiff muscles and built-up scar tissue, thus reducing pain. Your teacher will arrange the props for you and make sure you are comfortable and feel deeply supported. Many patients tell me that restorative poses allow their body and mind to settle into a place of stillness and deep contentment as they rest quietly in the present moment and find peace within.

Chi Kung (Qigong) and Tai Chi

Chi Kung is an ancient Chinese health-care practice that integrates physical postures, breathing techniques, and focused attention. The gentle, rhythmic movements of both Chi Kung and Tai Chi reduce stress, build stamina, increase vitality, and enhance the immune system. The physical parts of the exercises are fairly mild and can be performed by anyone. If you have severely limited mobility or flexibility, modifications to the exercises can be adapted easily to your needs.

"I've had more than a few clients who were highly skeptical, even averse to Chi Kung who end up appreciating and benefiting from the exercises," explains Greg Pergament, a certified Chi Kung instructor who works with patients in chronic pain at Las Vegas Recovery Center and is the author of the book *Chi Kung in Recovery*. "By gently increasing flexibility so that clients can gradually improve mobility and function of simple movements like walking and balance, Chi Kung becomes a source of hope for people who have suffered so long with debilitating physical issues that the will to exercise was lost. Restoring hope has been the most pronounced benefit of my Chi Kung work."

Greg offers the following testimonials from patients who have participated in his classes:

- "I didn't want to do it at first but now I love it."
- "I feel better every time I do Chi Kung."
- "My pain decreases when I am doing Chi Kung."
- "My dizziness and balance issues have stopped."
- "I feel like I have more energy after Chi Kung."
- "Chi Kung makes me feel more alive."

SLEEP

Sleep is the trump card . . . not sleeping well is
not an option in the successful treatment of chronic pain.

—DAVID HANSCOM, MD

A good night's sleep is critically important for people with chronic pain. If you sleep well at night, you will feel calmer and more relaxed during the day. I developed the following fifteen tips for a good night's sleep, which have proven to be a great help for me and for my patients as well. You don't have to incorporate all the points into your daytime and nighttime rituals, but be aware that there are many different strategies you can utilize to get a good night's sleep. If one particular approach doesn't appeal to you or work for you, try a different strategy or set of strategies. It may take a while to find the right formula for you—and you may have to give up some old habits (that lumpy childhood pillow or falling asleep with the TV on, for example)—so keep at it, please. Your aching body will really benefit from a good night's sleep!

1. **Nap during the day—judiciously!** Experts are divided on this one. If you are dealing with a lot of pain during the day, a short nap (ten to thirty minutes), or even just closing your eyes for five minutes may give you a dose of much-needed relaxation and energy. However, long naps may interfere with nighttime sleeping, especially the most restful and restorative stages of deep sleep and REM (rapid eye movement) sleep. If you nap regularly, I believe the best time is around two or three p.m., as short naps during this time are less likely to interfere with nighttime sleep. If you find that you are restless or waking up often at night, my recommendation is no naps until you are sleeping better and more consistently.

2. **Exercise during the day.** Exercise is vitally important but *when* and *how strenuously* you exercise may affect your sleep. Moderate to high-intensity exercise tends to increase circulating levels of the stress hormone cortisol, which will interfere with sleep, whereas low-intensity exercise will decrease cortisone levels, which will help you sleep. Thus, a slow walk around the block before bed may help you fall asleep and stay asleep, whereas running a mile may make it difficult to sleep. If you exercise strenuously, do it during the early part of your day, preferably before four p.m.

3. **Schedule a worry time.** It seems that when our brain is tired and ready for sleep, worries invariably creep into our consciousness. If you are prone to worrying, set time aside well before you go to bed to reflect on thoughts or experiences that are bothering you. Talking about your worries can help, as can writing them down in a journal (getting them off your mind and onto paper) or free-writing, which you toss away (along with your nagging, constantly circulating thoughts). For me, the worst time for worrying about something (anything!) is around three a.m. when I have to go to work the next day. If that's your pattern too, get out of bed and do something to relax (read a book, listen to a

relaxation CD, write in your journal) so you can let go of the thoughts, fears, and anxiety.

4. **Avoid caffeine, alcohol, and nicotine.** I can give you lots of reasons to avoid or eliminate these substances, but let me just say here that all three will interfere with your sleep. A good rule of thumb is no caffeine after noon and no alcohol or nicotine at least three hours before you go to bed. Of course, smokers tend to light up a cigarette when they can't sleep—a pattern I strongly encourage you to break. If sleeping is a big problem for you, I urge you to eliminate these stimulants all together.

5. **Lighten up on dinner and after-dinner snacks.** A heavy meal at dinner, especially carbohydrates, makes your body work hard to digest and process all that food. If you tend to eat late (after six p.m.), you may find it difficult to fall or stay asleep as your body is busy digesting the food. Go light and sleep tight. If you need a snack, have a cup of hot chamomile tea, a glass of warm milk, or a slice of tryptophan-rich turkey. (Tryptophan is an essential amino acid with a natural sedative effect.)

6. **Balance fluid intake.** Drink lots of water during the day. However, it's a good idea to limit your fluid intake a few hours before bedtime, lest you find that you have to get up in the middle of the night to use the bathroom and then have trouble falling back to sleep.

7. **Practice mindfulness-based stress reduction.** Try meditating before bed. Do the body scan exercise (page 179). Stretch and then rest in Shavasana (page 182). Or listen to a sleep-inducing CD (see the Resources section for recommendations).

8. **Avoid hot baths before bed.** Hot baths are relaxing but your body temperature needs to cool down in order to fall asleep—so, if you love hot baths, take one at least an hour before you go to bed. Hot packs on your neck and shoulders won't heat up your whole body and may help you relax before sleep.

9. **Keep cool while you sleep.** For most people, 65° to 70°F is ideal for nighttime sleep. If noise is not a problem, leave your window open for ventilation or use a fan (or air-conditioning during hot summer days). Fans also do double duty as noise blockers, similar to white noise machines. (See my next suggestion.)

10. **Block out noise.** You wouldn't believe how many people who have trouble sleeping find that their problems are miraculously cured with a white noise machine. (Earplugs will also do the trick, but they can be annoying and fall out.) The Marpac Dohm "sound conditioner" is a great choice and, although spendy, it is so well made that it should last for years. You can also download apps to help you sleep.

11. **Invest in quality pillows and mattresses.** A pillow or mattress that is too hard or too soft, too lumpy, too old, or too musty will not make bedtime a happy time. Investing in a good mattress and pillow is money well spent—just try out different types and brands to find what suits you best. Tempurpedic mattresses and mattress toppers work for some people, pillowtops for others, and firm mattresses for still others.

12. **Keep pen and paper next to your bed.** I often wake up with worrisome ideas or thoughts circling through my brain; writing them down allows me to dump them and free my mind. If nagging thoughts keep you awake, be sure to keep a pen and notebook by your bed and write down what's bugging you. When you wake up (refreshed after a good night's sleep, I hope), you might have your whole day's to-do list written out for you!

13. **Darken the room.** Light flooding into your room is a virtual alarm clock, telling you it's time to get up and get going. Avoid streetlights, your neighbors' floodlights, or early-morning sunshine by using room-darkening shades or blinds. You can also use a sleep mask, although some people find them uncomfortable. Another trick is to turn your alarm clock away from you. Most clocks emit light and some make a barely perceptible noise when the minutes change.

14. **Use your bed only for sleep (and sex).** So, get rid of the television, telephone, and computer! Reading a book of poetry or a literary work (not heart-thumpers, such as Stephen King or James Patterson novels) may be a good sleep inducer.

15. **Keep a consistent sleep schedule.** Some people ("larks") go to bed early and get up at first light. Others ("owls") like to stay up past midnight and sleep in. Gene variants may determine your particular sleep pattern, so trying to adjust to a different schedule can be difficult. No matter what, though, it's important to

get at least six and preferably eight hours of sleep at night. The key is to sleep and wake up at the same time every day (which may be impossible, of course, if you work a split shift, have a job where you are on call, or have young children in the house). But do the best you can, using these fifteen tips, to get a good night's sleep.

NUTRITION

What you eat and drink—and the dietary supplements you take—will have a profound impact on your pain levels. As Neil Barnard, MD, writes in the tremendously helpful *Foods That Fight Pain*:

> Nutrients work against pain in four ways. They can reduce damage at the site of injury, cool your body's inflammatory response, provide analgesia on pain nerves themselves, and even work within the brain to reduce pain sensitivity.

Nutrition is so important that we have devoted an entire chapter to this topic. See Chapter 10 for general nutritional guidelines to help reduce chronic pain, along with dietary recommendations; and see the Appendix, pages 265–292, for recipes to help you get started.

TOXINS

Toxins are any substance (natural or man-made) that can damage your body (and therefore your mind and spirit), exacerbate your pain, and cause or accelerate disease. Pesticides, medicines, emotions, and even certain people can be toxic and therefore deleterious to your health. The most notorious toxin, however, is from cigarettes—both tobacco smoke and nicotine are known to increase and intensify chronic pain, and secondhand smoke (from the lighted end of a cigarette, pipe, or cigar, or the smoke exhaled by a smoker) has high concentrations of cancer-causing agents that can increase pain, not to mention the greatly elevated risk of cancer and respiratory illnesses.

I'm convinced that of all the offending toxins in our world, tobacco smoke is the worst. I really hate it—because I know that smoking cigarettes or cigars or chewing tobacco truly harms my patients. I know that

Before Taking Supplements . . .

More than half of all Americans take one or more dietary supplements daily or on occasion, according to the National Institutes of Health (NIH). While it's possible to get all the nutrients you need from a healthy, balanced diet, your health-care practitioner may recommend a vitamin or mineral supplement or an herbal product (also known as botanicals).

Because some supplements may have side effects, especially when combined with other medications, be sure to talk to your doctor before taking supplements. It's also important to note that supplements will not cure, treat, or prevent chronic pain, although certain supplements may enhance your health and well-being.

Learn about the potential benefits and risks before taking dietary supplements by speaking to a health-care provider who is familiar with these products (perhaps your acupuncturist, homeopath, chiropractor, or massage therapist has such expertise). You can also find reliable information and fact sheets on dietary supplements at the National Institutes of Health website, and NIH recently launched a free online Dietary Supplement Label Database that lists the ingredients of thousands of dietary supplements and includes information on dosage, health claims, and cautions.

In general, I recommend the following vitamins and dosages, but *always* check with your health-care provider before taking any supplement because of the potential for side effects and interactions with medications you may be taking.

Vitamin D regulates inflammation throughout the body and supports our immune system: 2,000 IU of vitamin D_3 per day is a recommended dose, but some suggest up to 5,000 IU per day, especially if sunlight is in short supply.

Magnesium is an effective muscle relaxant that is particularly important for arthritic conditions, as it allows calcium to bond into the bone: 500–1,000 mg daily (choose a supplement that is "chelated with amino acids").

Fish oil supplements contain anti-inflammatory omega-3 fatty acids, specifically EPA (eicosapentaenoic acid) and DHA (docosahexaenoic acid). A good balance is 700–1,000 mg of EPA and 200–500 mg of DHA daily.

to quit smoking (or stop chewing tobacco) really does make people with chronic pain feel better.

And I also know that, of all addictions, nicotine may be one of the toughest to quit. Many experts—along with people who have quit using heroin or alcohol but have a significantly tougher time kicking their nicotine addiction—conclude that quitting smoking is the hardest addiction of all to break. About 90 percent of smokers who try to quit will relapse. Does that mean "Why bother"? Not at all, for it's a fact that everyone who has successfully quit has relapsed several times in the past. If you've tried to quit but started smoking (or chewing) again: "Keep trying!" and "Try harder!"

Researchers recently uncovered a neurological explanation for nicotine's tenacious grip—the nicotine withdrawal syndrome basically knocks out the power line that allows the brain to switch from the "default mode" brain network to the "executive control" network. Smokers in withdrawal are stuck in the "all about me" mode (also called the introspective, or self-referential, state) and can't make the leap to the self-restraint, or executive control, mode. While the post-acute withdrawal period (which lasts for months, even years) is often difficult for people with addictions to other drugs as well, smokers seem to be affected more intensely.

"Smokers who quit have a more difficult time shifting gears from inward thoughts about how they feel to an outward focus on the tasks at hand," says Dr. Caryn Lerman of the University of Pennsylvania's new Brain Behavior Laboratory. Smoked nicotine molecules reach the brain within seconds, where they grab hold of receptors on brain cells, rapidly releasing waves of dopamine and other feel-good chemicals. As you continue to smoke and smoke more and more often, your brain cells will produce more nicotine receptors. The more receptors, the greater the craving, and the tougher it is to cut back or quit. Anyone who has tried to cut back or stop smoking knows what I am talking about (and that includes both me and Kathy, as we both quit over thirty-five years ago). However, I will make you this promise: When you quit smoking or stop chewing, your pain will diminish.

Research leaves no doubt that the poisons in nicotine are directly related to increased pain. Studies show that smoking alters the body's absorption, distribution, and metabolism of opioids, so that smokers tend to use more opioid drugs than nonsmokers and yet report greater pain. So, if you are a smoker, you will likely use more painkilling drugs but experience *more* pain.

And here are more striking, eye-opening facts about smoking and chronic pain: Longitudinal studies show a relationship between the number of cigarettes smoked and the development of back pain. According to a recent study, people with low back pain and lumbar disk disease have significantly less pain when they quit smoking. Smokers with fibromyalgia miss more days of work, experience greater anxiety and depression and sleep disturbances, and report more pain, stiffness, and fatigue than nonsmokers do. Researchers hypothesize that smoking may speed up degenerative changes (from osteoporosis and lumbar disk disease, for example) and impair bone healing, thus slowing down healing, predisposing the smoker to injury, and increasing the risk of chronic pain. Smokers have higher rates of mood disorders such as depression and anxiety.

Nicotine does have analgesic properties—which is part of its draw—that can reduce the smoker's perception of pain for several seconds or at most a few minutes. Thus the "acute" effect of smoking may include a very brief period of pain relief, but the cost of that momentary reprieve, as the research clearly shows, is almost certainly more chronic pain. And, of course, we cannot forget the very real risks of cancer and lung disease.

Weigh the risks. Consider the painful, long-term impact and rationally balance it against the very brief pleasure of puffing on a cigarette. I hope you will heed this simple advice: If you smoke—get help and stop. There are helpful ways to quit and organizations to support you when you decide to do so. Several are listed in the Resources section. Quitting can be facilitated by patches and gum (while remembering that they also contain nicotine) and two medications: Zyban and Chantix. These methods may help you quit successfully, so be sure to ask your doctor for advice and guidance.

And of course, if you don't smoke—never start.

> If you smoke, quit.
> If you don't smoke—never start.

A word about e-cigarettes: The concentrated nicotine juice in these battery-operated devices is anything but safe. Although aggressively marketed by manufacturers as harmless or "relatively harmless" compared to cigarette smoking, recent research shows that "vaping" (inhaling the liquid solution of nicotine and flavors) causes you to inhale tiny particles that can irritate lung tissue and cause disease. Some e-cigarette models allow the user to adjust the voltage that heats up the liquid nicotine, intensifying the effect of the nicotine hit and converting chemical solvents in the e-liquid into formaldehyde and acetaldehyde, both of which are considered highly toxic.

ACUPRESSURE/ACUPUNCTURE

Thousands of years ago the Chinese developed a map of the human body, identifying sixteen invisible channels (meridians) through which our internal energy (chi) flows. Along these meridians, like cities on a highway map, are 365 acupuncture points (also called acupoints), many of which correspond to internal organs and other areas of the external body. By needling (acupuncture), or massaging or pressing (acupressure) these points, you can influence the energy flowing through your body, thereby reducing inflammation and pain.

The following acupoints are easy to locate and massage or press yourself. Use your thumb or fingers to massage the point in small, circular movements, always moving in a clockwise direction. Continue for two or three minutes and repeat several times a day. When pressing or stimulating these points, try hard to be "intentional"—concentrate, focus inward, and be purposeful as you imagine the energy moving freely again, resolving blockages throughout your body to restore flow and relieve pain. Pressure and intent work hand in hand. If you can visualize the flow of energy and believe you are healing yourself—you are.

- **Large Intestine 4 ("Great Eliminator" or "Joining of the Valleys")** is known as "the pain point"—when you feel pain anywhere in the body, use LI4. Acupuncturists often use this point for dispersing energy that is "stuck" in the upper part of the body, particularly the head and neck area, and for relieving headaches, sinus congestion, neck or shoulder tightness with pain and spasm.

Pressing or massaging this point will also help soothe your digestive system, alleviating gas, diarrhea, and constipation. LI4 is located on the top of the hand, in the webbing between the thumb and index finger.

- **Liver 3 ("Great Rushing")** can help with tremors, muscle twitches, migrating pains, dizziness, headaches, and digestive problems associated with stress. Liver 3 is located on the upper part of the foot, in the depression in the webbing between the big toe and the second toe.

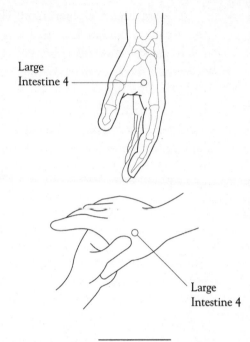

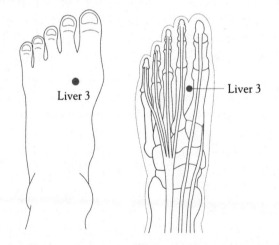

Note: Acupuncturists often use Large Intestine 4 and Liver 3 together, stimulating each point on both sides of the body to open the "Four Gates," releasing "stuck" energy and stagnation. When these four points are stimulated, imagine that the "windows" of your body are flung open, letting fresh air flow in, flooding the system with pure energy, and resolving painful obstructions.

- **Kidney 3 ("Great Mountain Stream")** is often used to relieve low back pain, knee pain, urinary incontinence, and lack of sexual vigor and/or interest; it is also effective for agitation, hot flashes, night sweats, insomnia, restless sleep, or itchy, irritated eyes. Kidney 3 is located in the depression between the inside ankle bone and the Achilles tendon. Use your fingers to put mild pressure in the valley until you feel the tender spot.

Kidney 3

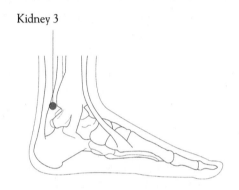

- **Conception Vessel 4 ("Sea of Chi, Sea of Energy")** is often called the *tantien* or "center point" and is said to connect directly to the Kidney chi reserves, which are used to ignite and sustain all the body's functions. Some acupuncturists call this point "Life Gate Fire" because of its ability to relieve fatigue and exhaustion, enhance immune function, rekindle sexual energies, and promote general well-being. CV4 is located on the midline of the lower belly, halfway between your belly button and your pubic bone. Lying down on your back, use your thumb or fingers to gently massage this point.

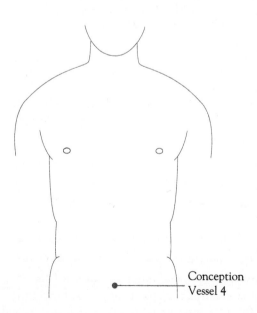

Conception Vessel 4

PROFESSIONAL THERAPIES

Dozens of professional therapies—techniques and strategies practiced by qualified, trained therapists—have been proven to help reduce chronic pain. Depending on your financial situation, insurance coverage, and individual preferences for specific approaches to pain reduction, the following methods can work wonders if you are open and willing to trying them. If you do want to investigate these healing methods, I recommend trying one modality at a time for a few weeks. Select the technique that appeals most to you before moving on to, or adding, another. Some patients discover a particular therapy that helps right away and they never feel the need to try others. Always do what works best for you. ("The Jump Start Plan" in Chapter 9 will help you in this process.)

ACUPUNCTURE: While you can easily put pressure on acupoints to relieve muscle tension, increase blood flow, and reduce chronic pain, as described on pages 155–157, it's always a good idea to spend at least a few sessions with a well-trained, skillful, and compassionate acupuncturist. Many of my patients get significant relief from pain with this treatment, which dates back thousands of years. The acupuncturist inserts hair-thin steel needles into the body at predetermined points to unblock and stimulate the energy (chi) channels. Researchers believe acupuncture relieves pain by increasing the release of endorphins. Patients report good results in relief of back and neck pain, muscle pain, headache, facial pain, arthritis, shingles, and many other conditions.

My brother and close friend, Larry, is just one person who's had great success with acupuncture: "I have arthritis in a number of areas—hands, wrists, knees, elbows, and so forth—which would potentially cause me a lot of pain and issues if I did not do maintenance. Many of the treatment areas have removed the pain completely and other areas keep it controlled. A few of the points in my head and ears are for relaxation, which is also beneficial. I am a very practical person and as long as I'm there, I figure I might as well cover all those areas!"

PHYSICAL THERAPY is the evaluation and treatment of musculoskeletal and neuromuscular disorders and pathologies. The goal is to restore functional movement, improve strength, and reduce pain. Practitioners believe functional movement is essential for good health, and I certainly concur. Find a therapist who will work with you to determine your individual treatment needs and goals. Your physical therapist may use "passive therapies," including traction, electrical muscle stimulation, hot and cold packs, moist heat, and ultrasound to increase blood flow, tissue relaxation, and breakdown of scar tissue. Manual therapies involving soft tissue and joint mobilization are especially effective in treating chronic pain and restoring full mobility. "Active therapies" help chronic pain patients take control of their pain and include strengthening exercises, stretching, and aerobic conditioning.

"The patient with chronic pain will be evaluated and a treatment plan will be established based on test findings, the patient's tolerance, and the patient's goals," explains physical therapist George Arias. "Appropriate exercise is emphasized due to the many positive physiological effects derived from movement, flexibility, and improved strength. Because patients directly and actively participate in their treatment and help determine the course of therapy, they gain a sense of control over the outcome."

CHIROPRACTIC THERAPY usually involves spinal manipulation (also called spinal adjustment) that uses pressure on the joint to improve pain and function. Careful, controlled manipulation can be done with the hands or a special device with the goal of increasing movement in the joint, relaxing the muscles, easing pain, and supporting the body's natural ability to heal itself. Chiropractic treatments also may involve heat and ice, electrical stimulation, relaxation techniques, and dietary supplements and recommendations. Research shows that chiropractic medicine is effective in many cases to reduce and treat acute and chronic back pain, and it also may be helpful for painful conditions, such as frozen shoulder, muscle spasms, carpal tunnel syndrome, among others.

Once again, "gentle" is the key word, as chiropractor Rich Bakir, who has worked with patients at LVRC for years, explains: "I always err on the side of too gentle and work toward more movement-based techniques, establishing trust and rapport with the patient and gauging their pain tolerances and sensitivity. This also gives me a baseline to work from as far as muscle spasms, vertebrae misalignment, hypertonicity (increased muscle tone usually indicating a problem area), and any radiation of pain. It's important to treat the chronic pain patient as a whole, not as an individual section or area of pain and discomfort."

TENS (**transcutaneous electrical nerve stimulation**) is sometimes described as the electrical equivalent of portable acupuncture or acupressure. TENS units are small, battery-powered devices about the size of a cell phone. They generate a small electrical current, delivered through electrodes or patches placed on the skin, intended to override or block pain signals from the nerves to the spinal cord or brain. (A surgeon can also place the electrodes beneath the skin with an implantable spinal cord stimulator.) You use a switch to control the strength of the electrical impulse, which is not painful (except at high levels), although the "pins and needles" sensation can be annoying for some people. Although you can use the TENS unit at home, be sure to ask your doctor or therapist for professional guidance on how to use the unit safely and effectively.

I have a TENS unit that I use when my back is acting up on a high-pain day. I hook up the electrodes and lie down for twenty or thirty minutes. The pulsations leave me feeling less tight and more relaxed and invariably reduce my pain level. When she developed a spinal headache (often described as "a headache like no other") after an epidural anesthetic during the birth of her second child, Kathy used a TENS unit for several weeks. "The doctors couldn't stop the spinal leak," Kathy told me, "and the pain was excruciating. The TENS unit helped me bear the pain."

Many medical supply companies will give you a "loaner" model to try out before you buy the unit, or ask your physical therapist or chiropractor if they loan or sell TENS units. If you are insured, insurance companies often cover the cost.

MASSAGE increases the flow of blood and oxygen to specific areas of the body, relaxing and warming the soft tissues, and decreasing pain through gentle or firm pressure, friction movements that go across the grain of the muscles, and light or deep touch. There's nothing like being touched since so many of us with chronic pain are truly touch-deprived. You can choose from dozens of different varieties of massage, and every massage practitioner brings his or her own style, technique, and energy to the process. It's not uncommon for patients to try different massage methods and switch masseuses before they find someone with whom they feel completely comfortable and whose technique is just right for their needs. Here are a few tried-and-true methods that you might investigate:

- Swedish massage, in which the massage therapist uses kneading, friction, and long strokes on the muscles and joints to increase relaxation and flexibility
- Deep-tissue massage, in which the therapist uses strokes and pressure on different muscles of the body, focusing on deep rather than superficial muscle groups
- Pressure-point massage in which the therapist applies focused pressure on myofascial (*myo* refers to muscle and *fascial* refers to connective tissue) trigger points—the junctions between the muscles and the connective tissue, and uncomfortable points or knots that form in the body
- Rolfing uses techniques that seek to realign your body by targeting the connective tissue (myofascia) that surrounds your muscles. Poor posture is often one source of headaches, backaches, and joint pain, and Rolfing can be a very effective technique for realigning your posture. Many people find the treatments helpful, but be aware that Rolfing is a deep, rather forceful massage method. If you are interested in investigating Rolfing, find a local practitioner and ask about their technique and treatment philosophy for people in chronic pain. Perhaps try a session and then make a decision about whether this particular treatment method is for you.

AYURVEDA is an ancient art and science dating back five thousand years. The goal of Ayurveda (which means "the science of life") is to restore balance through a healthy lifestyle and diet, physical exertion, and proper nutrition and digestion. According to the Chopra Center, founded in 1996 by Deepak Chopra, MD, and David Simon, MD, Ayurvedic medicine seeks to identify an individual's "ideal state of balance, determine where they are out of balance, and offer interventions using diet, herbs, aromatherapy, massage treatments, music, and meditation to reestablish balance."

Imbalances that cause or contribute to chronic pain include toxins that accumulate in our tissues and block circulation, poor nutrition, poor digestion, nervous system imbalances, physical and mental stress, immune system dysfunction, and disturbances in our natural biological rhythms. Ayurvedic practitioners seek to invigorate the body's natural ability to heal and repair itself, using therapies that include herbalized oil massage, proper food nutrition and food preparation, meditation, herbs, yoga positions, and yoga breathing exercises.

HYDROTHERAPY (water therapy) can be very effective for chronic pain relief. Cold therapy helps to relieve painful swelling and reduce inflammation by slowing down blood flow to the area, which also slows down pain messages from your nerves to your brain. Heat therapy alleviates pain and stiffness by increasing circulation and blood flow and helping your muscles relax. Water therapy is often used for back and neck pain, arthritis, fibromyalgia, and other joint pain. Trained hydrotherapists will guide you in using Hubbard tank and whirlpool therapy, as well as offering guidelines to most effectively use sitz baths and suggesting exercises you can do in swimming pools. Showers and baths, of course, do not require professional guidance!

> **Hubbard tank:** You immerse your entire body in this large, industrial whirlpool, and the warm, gently agitated water helps increase blood circulation, decrease stress on bones and joints, and reduce swelling. The massaging effect of the warm water can be very helpful for muscle strains and spasms as well as easing the pain of arthritic conditions.
>
> **Whirlpool therapy** uses heated churning water to ease aching muscles, help chronic spinal conditions, and induce relaxation.
>
> **Sitz baths**, in which you sit in a small tub with water up to the hips, are used to relieve discomfort and pain in the lower part of the body, including lumbar (low back) pain, pelvic pain, prostate infections (prostatitis), rectal, and testicular pain.
>
> **Swimming pools:** Water provides buoyancy to support your body and resistance to help build strength and endurance. Low-impact exercises are particularly beneficial for people with chronic pain.
>
> **Showers and baths** are truly one of the minor miracles of the modern world. Most of us tend to get into the routine of taking a shower in the morning when we wake up, but if you are feeling stressed and anxious, taking the time to stand in a warm or hot shower or relax in your bathtub (or an outdoor hot tub) at any time of day can be truly healing.

REIKI is a Japanese technique used for stress reduction and relaxation. "Reiki is a very specific form of energy healing, in which hands are placed just off the body or lightly touching the body," according to the Johns Hopkins Integrative Medicine and Digestive Center. "The intention is to create deep relaxation, to help speed healing, reduce pain, and decrease other symptoms you may be experiencing."

Cheryl, our yoga instructor, is also a Reiki Master who has often witnessed the healing that takes place during Reiki sessions. "Just about everyone I have worked on feels more relaxed after the session and even just the simple act of relaxing and feeling the support of another person drops pain levels," she explains. "Of course, the more receptive the patient is, the more benefits are received."

I'll never forget Horace, a Vermonter who was dead set against any "New Age fiddle-faddle," as he put it. He vehemently refused to give Reiki a try until the day his roommate came out of a Reiki session looking calm and blissed out. So, into the therapy room seventy-year-old Horace went, and he told me later he was really impressed by the results. "My neck pain was gone—gone!—for a week after that first treatment," he exclaimed. Four years later, he is still working with a Reiki Master, driving ninety minutes each way for his sessions.

BIOFEEDBACK: In a biofeedback session, the therapist will connect a measuring device to record electrical potentials in the cerebral cortex (electroencephalography or EEG) or in the skeletal muscles (electromyography or EMG) to your skin. A computer collects the data, which are expressed in sound or by light waves (which you can see on the computer grid). Thermal biofeedback measures skin temperature, galvanic skin response indicates the amount of anxiety you may be experiencing, and peripheral skin temperature can be measured to assess stress levels. Based on the data collected, the therapist will suggest specific mental exercises designed to help you modify brain processes and muscle control, helping to lessen neck and back pain, headaches, and teeth grinding. While many people find biofeedback helpful (and research confirms its effectiveness), others have trouble mastering the techniques and do not experience relief from the procedure.

Ask your doctor or another health-care professional to recommend a biofeedback therapist who has experience working with people with chronic pain.

Aromatherapy, which uses essential oils distilled from plants, flowers, trees, bark, grasses, seeds, and fruits, dates back six thousand years. Imhotep (circa 2600–2500 BC), chancellor to the pharaoh and high priest to the Egyptian sun god Ra, used essential oils in massages, baths, and embalming of the dead. Hippocrates (460–370 BC), considered one of the most important figures in the history of medicine, used aromatherapy to rid Athens of the plague. Today aromatherapy is used for its anti-depressant, anti-viral, anti-inflammatory, and analgesic properties to treat a variety of ailments ranging from fatigue, tension, anxiety, depression, stress, and chronic pain. Massage therapists often use scented oils and candles to enhance the therapeutic experience.

Wintergreen, peppermint, lavender, spruce, marjoram, and sandalwood are among the most popular essential oils for relieving chronic pain. You can use them at home for hand or foot massages or when you press specific pain-relieving acupoints. I've had many patients tell me that they never travel without their scented candles, and others rave about their aromatherapy diffusers that they use in their homes and offices. Experimenting with the wide variety of these and other scents that are available—cedar, chamomile, eucalyptus, frankincense, grapefruit, jasmine, lemongrass, orange, vanilla—can be soothing, invigorating, and great fun.

OXYGEN THERAPY: Nerves are exquisitely sensitive to cellular oxygen levels, and even a tiny reduction in oxygen can cause numbness, pain, tingling, and weakness. The best, easiest, and cheapest form of oxygen therapy (and the one I recommend to all my patients) is proper breathing. I will discuss different breathing techniques in detail in the next chapter. Yoga, meditation, Tai Chi, and Chi Kung are all forms of "oxygen therapy," relying on focused breathing techniques that have the added benefit of boosting your circulation and the oxygen content of your tissues (oxygen boost). Regularly practicing deep breathing exercises increase the elasticity of blood vessels by gently increasing the pressure within them, causing the capillaries to flood with oxygen-carrying blood—but without increasing pressure on the heart to work harder to boost circulation.

Mental, physical, and emotional balance are intricately interconnected and interdependent. In the next chapter you will find many helpful steps and strategies to help reduce negative emotional states and increase the frequency and intensity of positive emotions.

SEVEN

REGAINING EMOTIONAL EQUILIBRIUM
Balancing Your Emotions with Mindfulness

People who are habitually mindful of their current
experiences are more likely to experience frequent and
intense positive emotions, to feel self-sufficient
and competent, and to have positive social relationships.

—SONJA LYUBOMIRSKY, *THE HOW OF HAPPINESS*

Attaining and maintaining emotional balance is difficult for
all human beings, but people living with chronic pain have additional
challenges. Many of us tend to push our emotions deep inside, bury-
ing and negating them, trying to convince ourselves that our feelings
aren't valid or, worse, that we have no feelings and simply "don't care,"
because the emotions we are experiencing are just too strong, too negative, too overwhelming. I can't tell you how many people have told me
in our first or second meeting, "I'm not angry; I forgot all about that,"
or "It's in the past and I don't think of it," only to be overcome with
deep emotional distress when the topic is brought up later in group or
in a one-on-one session.

Emotions are such a big part of the overall experience of chronic
pain that I believe it is imperative for you to dive into this chapter
with all the earnestness you can muster. The breathing exercises and
mindfulness practices detailed in these pages can truly turn your life
around. Gaining a foothold on how your emotions affect you, learning
to reduce the stress you feel, and freeing yourself from the bonds of

thoughts and feelings that have dominated your existence for months, years, even decades will enable you to free yourself from these tenacious emotional hooks.

Andy, 39, is a perfect example. He was so tired of living with the anger, guilt, and fear of the past—he was repeatedly physically and sexually abused by his fourth grade teacher—that he willingly rummaged through his memories of the past, bringing them to light, and working through the shame he lived with every day. After a few weeks in treatment, he began to make the connection between his strong emotions and his debilitating migraine headaches. He talked openly and honestly about the awareness he was having regarding his childhood and how those early experiences sabotaged his current relationships and distorted his sense of self, and the more he talked (as tough as it was), the less his head hurt.

My dear friends Sharon Wegscheider-Cruse and Joe Cruse first coined the term *emotional abscess*, drawing an analogy between buried emotions and an abscess deep in your gut, walled off and full of infection. The septic tissue is invisible and hurts only if you bump or press against it, but it is always leaking, poisoning you, making you feel feverish and achy. Proper treatment of an abscess is to puncture it and safely drain out the infected material. It's the same with those buried feelings. If you don't unearth your buried emotions and then clear them out, they will continue to contaminate your very existence, making you hurt more. This takes time, patience, and healing from the inside out.

The word *should* comes up often in our experiences with chronic pain. "I should be strong." "I shouldn't be so angry and resentful." "He should pay more attention to me." "She should be a better friend." All those *shoulds* sink a spade into the earth of our memories where we try to bury the emotions we "shouldn't" feel, and then cover them up with thick layers of dirt and clay. But the groundwater of bitterness and resentment seep out, for living with a chorus of *shoulds* never works.

Sometimes we go to the opposite extreme and aggressively fight for our rights, engaging in angry, bitter battles with our doctors, coworkers, friends, family members, and even strangers. Aggressive tailgaters are my nemesis. I often get the urge to slam on my brakes. We also fight with and against ourselves. "I'm so sick and tired of my husband's martyred expressions," Joanna said bitterly. "If my life is such a burden to him, he should just leave me and find a healthy new wife."

"Everyone is picking on me in group," Riley grumbled. "It's the same old story; no one likes me because I'm so difficult."

MINDFULNESS

Where is the balance between hiding your emotions and over-exposing them, resulting in a feeling of being overwhelmed? In this chapter I will focus on mindfulness practices and techniques that will help you navigate through difficult and demanding emotional terrain. Perhaps the most challenging landscape of all is the shame and dislike you may have for the parts of your body that are in pain. "My arthritic fingers are so gnarled and inflamed that it disgusts me just to look at them." "Scoliosis has twisted and distorted my spine to the point that I can't stand to look at myself in the mirror." Shame may distort your entire sense of self as you judge yourself to be "unattractive," "undesirable," "weakly," "broken down," and "unlovable."

Mindfulness will help you become more aware of shameful thoughts and knee-jerk reactions. The words of Jon Kabat-Zinn capture both the practical application and the spiritual essence of the term:

> In Asian languages, the word for *mind* and the word for *heart* are same. So if you're not hearing mindfulness in some deep way as heartfulness, you're not really understanding it. Compassion and kindness towards oneself are intrinsically woven into it. You could think of mindfulness as wise and affectionate attention.

Once again I am reminded of Jon's words in his book *Full Catastrophe Living*: "As long as you are breathing, there is more right with you than wrong with you, no matter what is wrong." I sincerely hope that the strategies and techniques described in the remainder of this chapter help you to understand and internalize Jon Kabat-Zinn's profound observation as it applies to you and your life. These exercises are intended to put you in touch with your authentic self, allow you to see and understand your thoughts and emotions nonjudgmentally, and guide you to connect with other people and the world itself in ways that enlarge and expand rather than constrict and contract. We spend far too much time, in our head, looking at (and searching for) what is wrong with ourselves, others, and the world we inhabit—and that negative, self-critical, and world-weary focus directly impacts the depth and intensity of our chronic pain and our overall physical health. Critical thoughts and feelings, stemming from a universal sense of unworthiness, can begin to dominate our essence—unless we do something to change.

Isn't it time for us to discover a new way of looking and seeing, acknowledging and accepting what is "right" with us and our world? I'm not talking about positive thinking or suggesting that you cheerfully repeat affirmations like the character named Stuart from *Saturday Night Live* does ("I'm good enough, I'm smart enough, and doggone it, people like me!"). Seriously, when you're in pain, why and how would you want to put up with such platitudes, especially when they are, at least in the moment, so patently untrue?

Both unbridled optimism and unregulated pessimism are equally misguided. As writer Barbara Ehrenreich discusses in a *Time* magazine post titled "The Peril of Positive Thinking":

> What we need here is some realism, or the simple admission that, to paraphrase a bumper sticker, "stuff happens," including sometimes very, very bad stuff. We don't have to dwell incessantly on the worst-case scenarios—the metastasis, the market crash or global pandemic—but we do need to acknowledge that they could happen and prepare in the best way we can. Some will call this negative thinking, but the technical term is sobriety.
>
> Besides, the constant effort of maintaining optimism in the face of considerable counterevidence is just too damn much work. Optimism training, affirmations and related forms of self-hypnosis are a burden that we can finally, in good conscience, set down. They won't make you richer or healthier, and, as we should have learned by now, they can easily put you in harm's way. The threats that we face, individually and collectively, won't be solved by wishful thinking but by a clear-eyed commitment to taking action in the world.

Taking action in the world begins with taking action in *your* world. There is no "goal" of mindfulness practices—just being present, as best you can, is the instruction. I work with many people who say "I can't meditate right" or "It doesn't work." Pema Chödrön advises: "Give up all hope of fruition." If you just engage in the process—and be curious and nonjudgmental about each moment—*that* is mindfulness meditation.

The first time I met with Patricia, 52, we were sitting in my office as I described mindfulness and the emotional aspects of pain. She looked up at my bookcase and with an eager expression pointed to a book and said, "I want this one—*Medication for Chronic Pain*."

"Actually, the title is *Meditation for Chronic Pain*," I said with a smile.

After we had a laugh, she stood up, somewhat stiffly because of the rheumatoid arthritis that inflamed her joints, took the book off the shelf, and said, "Okay, can I borrow this? I'm ready to get started."

Tangible, Immediate Benefits

Mindfulness exercises and meditation offer many tangible and immediate benefits. Hundreds of research studies show that practicing mindfulness, even for a short time, can be beneficial for your body, your mind, and your relationships. For example, mindfulness exercises:

- Enhance your immune system's ability to fight off illness and disease
- Increase the density of gray matter in areas of the brain linked to emotional regulation, learning, and memory
- Boost positive emotions while reducing negative emotions
- Reduce stress
- Fight depression
- Help you tune out distractions
- Improve your memory and ability to focus and pay attention
- Increase activity in the neurocircuitry involved in empathy and self-compassion
- Through fostering optimism and relaxation, help you feel more accepting of and connected to others
- Lead to healthier eating, exercise, and sleeping habits
- And of course—and perhaps best of all—these benefits lead directly to a reduction in physical pain.

I suggest that you read through the mindfulness exercises discussed in the remainder of this chapter and select the one(s) that are most appealing or meaningful to you. Practice for five or ten minutes every day. Then, when you are ready, try a different exercise. A week or two later, try another. After a month of experimenting, you will have built yourself a routine of mindfulness practices to integrate into your day. This may seem like a lot of "building," but here's the thing about mindfulness—once you pay attention and become aware of something, no matter how small or seemingly trivial, it can then become integrated into your normal routine. In other words, mindfulness becomes part of you, part of the way you live your life—not just part of your "doing" but part of your "being." Rather than dread these exercises as "yet one more thing to do today," the chances are very good that you will look forward to them, as I do, as one of the highlights of your day.

BREATHING

Deep Breathing

Deep breathing reminds us how important it is to just breathe, focusing our attention on the simple act of inhaling and exhaling—inhaling pure, invigorating oxygen and exhaling carbon dioxide and any toxins that might have built up in your body. Following, I list several simple deep breathing techniques that are perfect for beginners. Remember, you don't have to try them all. If you find just one that you can repeat every day for at least a week, begin there. Add in other techniques as your curiosity—and energy—allow. And please, be curious. Suspend your disbelief and give it your best shot.

Robert came to me in a very excited state. "You won't believe it, Doc! I don't believe it! I was sitting outside on a bench doing the breathing exercises I learned from my counselor and I felt a cool breeze across my body and my back pain *disappeared*. It's amazing!" he said, responding to the happy expression on my face. "For the first time in twenty years, I didn't feel pain in my back. And that was fifteen minutes ago and I'm still feeling pretty much pain-free! This stuff really works!"

I can promise you this: deep breathing exercises will increase your energy and make you feel better if you do them regularly. Recently, a middle-aged gentleman approached me after I gave a talk about the methods we teach patients at Las Vegas Recovery Center. "I'm filled with anxiety and in pain all the time, but I can't afford your fancy program," he said with a tinge of annoyance, even resentment in his voice. "I live on a fixed income. I'm not a Rockefeller, you know." My response was simple: "Your breath is available to you at no charge."

I suggested that he try to concentrate on his breathing when he was feeling anxious, because it is common to hold your breath or take shallow breaths. And I told him about the man who came to my office in excruciating pain (10 out of 10) who, after one minute of controlled breathing, relaxed and admitted that his pain dropped to a 4 out of 10.

"When you find your heart beating faster and your sense of frustration rising," I said, "you can purposefully slow your breathing and focus on the air moving in and out through your nostrils. Invariably you will find that your tension decreases and you will be able to handle the situation with equanimity."

My new friend nodded his head thoughtfully, shook my hand, and said, "Well, I appreciate this good advice—and it's free, too!"

The following breathing techniques are simple ways to practice noticing your breath going in and out. A few simple tips:

- The exercises can be done either sitting or lying down, however you are most comfortable. If you're lying down, though, you're more likely to fall asleep, and the keys to mindfulness are focused attention and awareness!
- Inhale through your nose.
- Exhale through your mouth with your lips slightly parted. No sound is necessary (except with the *om* exercise), although some people find that a soft "ah" as they exhale is soothing and a helpful reminder of the process.
- Keep the tip of your tongue on the ridge of tissue between your teeth and the roof of your mouth. This helps you keep your focus and remain calm and centered. Traditional Chinese Medicine practitioners believe the calming energy flow is created by stimulating the two "Master Meridians"—the Central Vessel, which ends at the tip of your tongue, and the Governing Vessel, which ends at the roof of your mouth.
- As you breathe, try not to exaggerate either the inhale or the exhale; just naturally fill your lungs and empty them, fill and empty, fill and empty.

- Repeat the exercise three to four times, and of course, continue for as long as you like. It's a good practice to add a few breaths each time you sit, if that feels okay.

Belly Breath

A traditional yoga breathing exercise, Bhastrika or the Bellows Breath works wonders for invigorating your body and mind with extra energy and vitality.

- Keeping your mouth closed but relaxed, breathe in and out rapidly through your nose, concentrating on fast, mechanical breathing similar to a bellows pumping air. The breath should be audible on both inhalation and exhalation. The inhalation and exhalation are equal in length and volume.
- Use your stomach (diaphragm) muscles to power the breath, contracting the belly muscles on exhalation and expanding the muscles on the inhalation. Rapid breathing is the goal, with as many as two or three inhalation/exhalation cycles per second.
- Begin with ten to fifteen seconds of rapid breathing, eventually working up to a full minute; repeat three or four times daily.
- End with a deep cleansing breath: Inhale fully through your nose, then exhale slowly through your mouth.

Calming Breath

When you are anxious, tense, or need to relax, try this breathing technique:

- Exhale completely through your mouth, then close your mouth and inhale through your nose to a count of five. As you breathe in, imagine that pure, clean air is entering your lungs.
- Hold your breath for ten counts, imagining that your cells are using this opportunity to empty their waste products into the bloodstream.
- Exhale to ten counts, visualizing the waste products exiting from your body.

Prana Breath

Prana means "life force" and pranayama is an ancient practice focusing on breath control. Research shows that pranayama can help relieve stress-related disorders, including anxiety and depression. The following exercise is sometimes referred to as the 6-3-6-3; repeat the 6-3-6-3 cycle several times, if you wish.

- Keeping your lips loosely together, inhale through your nose for six counts.
- Hold your breath for three counts.
- Exhale through your nose for six counts.
- Hold your breath for three counts.

Breathing Om

Om, or *Aum*, is a traditional Sanskrit mantra that is said to be the sound of the Earth moving through the Heavens since the beginning of time. What does *om* sound like? Cover your ears with the palms of your hands, listen carefully with your eyes closed, concentrate hard, and you can hear the blood moving through your capillaries—the blood whispers *om*. Put a seashell to your ear, and it's as if you can hear the ocean roar—the ocean says *om*. Listen to a gentle wind caressing a greening field of wheat—the wheat murmurs *om*.

Om may also be imagined as the sound beneath silence.

- Find a comfortable position with your back erect but not stiff. Place your hands on the upper part of your abdomen, about a hand's width above your navel.
- Breathe in deeply and when you exhale, say, "Ommmmmmmmmmmmmmm" continuing the sound for as long as possible without straining yourself. You may prefer to think of "singing" the *om*, adding melody as you like.
- When you are at the end of your breath, take another deep breath and say or sing, "Ommmmmmmmmmmmmmmmmm" again.
- Repeat this exercise for two to five minutes every day, varying the tone of the sounds as you like.

Rock On, Belly!

Massage therapist Lynda Christenson suggested this breathing exercise. Although it may seem a little strange at first, give it a try. The weight of the stone will feel soothing to your belly, and lifting the rock up and down as you breathe in and out is a bit like weight lifting with your abdominal and diaphragm muscles. Be sure to relax your upper chest muscles and use your diaphragm—the dome-shaped muscle that sits under your lungs—to do the work. Diaphragmatic breathing techniques will take some practicing, but ultimately, they will strengthen your "core"— the muscles that surround your vital organs, from your pelvic floor to your ribs and spine, wrapping around your body from back to front. A strong core enhances balance and stability, takes the pressure off your back muscles, helps with lower back pain, and strengthens your abdominal pelvic floor muscles (helping with incontinence and pelvic floor disorders, such as prolapse).

- Find a fairly large and not too heavy rock, approximately the size and weight of this book—come to think of it, you can use this book, if you want! Make sure the rock has a relatively flat surface on one side. You can usually find such rocks in rivers or stream beds, or you can purchase smooth, polished, extra-large massage stones on various Internet sites.
- Using your belly (diaphragm) muscles, breathe in and, as your abdomen rises, feel the rock elevate, too. Be careful not to use your back muscles—it's the belly that moves the rock!
- Hold your breath for five or ten seconds after you inhale, then use your diaphragm muscles to lower the rock on the exhalation.
- Lift and lower five to ten times. Repeat this gentle exercise several times a day.

MEDITATION

When Kathy and I first started working together on this book, I asked her whether she meditated. "It's on my to-do list," she responded, "but right now I'm too busy and stressed, I just don't have time."

She looked at me apologetically as if to say, "I know that's lame." We laughed and then I offered, "How about you just start with five minutes?"

Kathy started meditating that day and now she devotes ten to fifteen minutes every day to meditation, which she has discovered helps with her migraine headaches and shoulder and neck pain.

Meditation and mindfulness can begin for you right here, right now, with simple everyday activities. Imagine, for example, opening and closing your kitchen cabinets with focused attention on making no noise whatsoever, taking hold of the handle, slowly opening the cabinet door, gently removing a dish or a plate, then concentrating once again on closing the door little by little so that it shuts without a sound. I know that I've spent too much time in the past slamming doors in anger or frustration—car doors, front doors, back doors, office doors, bathroom doors—and, having made my point with great forcefulness, experienced remorse about disturbing the peace of others, not to mention my own peace of mind.

You may be a bit resistant to meditation, like Matt, 31, who refused to go to meditation class. When he met with his counselor, he said, "I can't meditate! All I can think about is my darn arm and hand pain and what this pain has done to my life. It's all so stupid—all this pain just because I fell off my bike and fractured my wrist!"

As they continued to talk, Matt revealed that he couldn't stop thinking about financial problems and things piling up at work while he was just "sitting there, doing nothing." The more he fretted about this and that, the more his arm and hand throbbed and ached.

"The point isn't to stop the mind," the counselor told him, "but to observe it. When you notice that your mind is wandering or racing, you are being mindful! Focus on your breath and allow thoughts and feelings to pass through without expectations of goals or outcomes. If your arm is screaming at you, simply notice that and focus your awareness without judgment and interpretations."

Matt listened attentively. "Okay, okay," he sighed, agreeing to try a short meditation exercise. Acknowledging the benefits of spending just a few minutes with his eyes closed, focusing on his breathing, he made a commitment to attend the next group session.

Everyday Contemplations

Everyday, in-the-moment contemplative exercises help ground us and steady our emotions. Just moving your neck from side to side, reaching up to the ceiling and stretching one side and then the other, walking to the mailbox, or taking a short stroll around the block offer time to focus on breathing. When you wake up in the morning or wash your hands after you go to the bathroom, you can mindfully pay attention to the everyday miracles that we all too often take for granted.

The short Jewish prayer *bracha* of *Asher Yatzar* celebrates mindfulness by honoring the marvelous complexity of the human body and its daily functioning. People living with chronic pain, especially those on opioids, will understand the relevance and deeper meaning of this prayer, for going to the bathroom can become one of life's most difficult endeavors. Jewish tradition asks that the prayer be recited every morning and again after using the bathroom. The blessing thanks Hashem (a common way to refer to God) for creating us with wisdom and including "many openings and many hollows . . . that if but one of them were to be ruptured or if one of them were to be blocked, it would be impossible to survive."

Mindfulness practices are simple, straightforward, stress-relieving, and potentially life changing. I like the way Jon Kabat-Zinn emphasizes that although mindfulness can be developed and nurtured through formal meditation, there are many ways of paying attention and cultivating a state of awareness and intimacy, not just with the self and not just with what knowingly lies outside the self, but with "spaciousness itself." In a Greater Good video titled "What Is Mindfulness?" Kabat-Zinn explains his basic philosophy:

> It's not really about sitting in the full lotus, like pretending you're a statue in a British museum. It's about living your life as if it really mattered, moment by moment by moment by moment.

All of this is to emphasize that there is no "right" way to be mindful. You don't have to attend a retreat, sit in a stiff posture for hours at a time, or seclude yourself in a dark room. Some people create a formal practice at a certain time of day for a specific number of minutes, but really all you need is five or ten minutes to be still and focus on your breathing "as if it *really mattered*, moment by moment by moment." Jon always adds "as best you can" in all his meditation instructions.

Caroline, 60, understood all about "as best you can," having endured seven surgeries for failed back syndrome and spinal stenosis. She sat calmly in the throes of her emotional turmoil, having just read a letter from her daughter lambasting her for being a terrible mother, caring more about her pain pills than her family. The tears subsided, she agreed to meet with her counselor, but she then asked whether she could take a few minutes to meditate. She wanted to calm her busy, defensive mind and settle down the rising headache and anxiety before she began the tough process of sorting out her feelings and responding to her angry daughter.

In the remainder of this chapter I will describe several mindfulness practices that work extremely well for people living with chronic pain. The Resources section on pages 293–296 includes a list of helpful books, websites, CDs, and DVDs, should you want to learn more about these powerful healing techniques.

The Body Scan

I met Andrea in the lunchroom as I arrived at the center one morning. She looked exhausted. "I woke up at two a.m. with abdominal cramping and diarrhea, just like I've always done for the last eight years," she said. "I despaired and decided this was never going to work and I should just as well be dead or back on my drugs, which at least would give me a few hours of sleep." I steeled myself for the next sentence and was delightfully surprised. "So, then I popped in the body scan CD you gave me," she said, "and believe it or not, my mind slowed down, the pain subsided, and I finally slept for a few hours. I feel better than I have in a long time."

After working with hundreds of patients in chronic pain, I am convinced that the body scan meditation is one of the most powerful mindfulness exercises available to us. Think of this meditation as getting to know your body nonjudgmentally. That's a powerful thought—how many of us thoroughly and intensely dislike parts of our body? Especially those of us with chronic pain? A classic story of feeling shame about his body and being in pain comes from Stan, a former athlete and Olympic skier who limped after a hip surgery and felt very self-conscious in sessions with the trainer. "I feel more like a Chevette than a Corvette," he told me. Stan is certainly not alone. Alana was miserable because of the "hunchback" she had developed due to severe osteoarthritis of her spine. Carl despised walking with a cane and, when he abandoned it too soon in his early recovery, ended up falling and seriously injuring his wrist. Karen would only wear loose clothing when she arrived in treatment, because of her swollen abdomen that was a direct result of constipation from the opioids.

All manner of unbecoming, unattractive, aching, and throbbing places may call forth your dislike and even contempt, undermining your sense of self and disrupting your emotional equilibrium. So, join with me in learning how to accept and, yes, like your body, feeling and appreciating each area that you focus on, letting go of the thoughts and judgments you traditionally have associated with specific body parts. Allow your thoughts and emotions to dissolve into a sense of timelessness, letting go and relaxing completely. At the same time, focus your attention on specific areas of your body that are calling out for your attention. Befriend those tender and scorned places for they are part of you, part of what makes you a unique and whole individual.

Focusing on the areas where you feel the most pain often helps disperse it. You can move the process along by breathing into the pain, much as a mother might blow gently on a child's wound. It is not the soft breath on a scrape or bruise that heals and makes whole again but the loving, undivided attention that another person bestows upon you, in this case your own attention on the painful areas. When you step back and observe the pain, the part of you that is observing is *not* in pain. Think about that!

The purpose of the body scan is not to relax or achieve a serene state of mind, although you may feel calm and at peace during and after the exercise. The goal of this practice is really about acceptance and being in the present moment, in the "right now."

We do body scans most days at the center—sometimes these sessions are run by staff and other times patients listen to a CD. Pain scores usually drop by 20 to 40 percent after these thirty- to forty-five-minute sessions. Here are some simple instructions:

Body Scan

1. Lie down on your back in a cozy, comfy place. Your bed is just fine, or you might have a yoga mat or foam pad that you could use on the floor.
2. If you tend to get cold, make sure you have a blanket nearby. Bolsters or pillows placed under your neck or knees may provide additional comfort.
3. Close your eyes if that feels relaxing and restful for you. Some people prefer to keep their eyes half-open, letting a little bit of light in so they don't fall asleep. (The body scan can also be used to induce sleep, but generally the point is to stay awake.)
4. Focus your attention on your belly. When you breathe in, feel your belly rise; when you breathe out, feel it fall.
5. Try to take deep, full breaths rather than short, shallow breaths. Some people like to lengthen the exhalation phase of the breathing rhythm, imagining that the "out" breath is a wave gently breaking on the shore, fully stretching itself before it recedes back into the ocean of the "in" breath.
6. For a minute or two, concentrate on your whole body, feeling the points of contact as your head, shoulders, elbows, hands, fingers, knees, thighs, ankles, and toes rest on the floor. If you are uncomfortable, adjust your body as necessary, and then settle back into a relaxed, open position.
7. Focus your awareness on the toes of your right foot. Imagine that your toes are breathing—this can take some practice! As you breathe in, think of the breath traveling through your bloodstream, carrying oxygen and essential nutrients from the tips of your toes to the top of your head. You may experience a need to wiggle your toes, which is just fine (and, of course, a smile doesn't hurt).
8. Focusing on your breathing, bring your awareness to another part of your body—calf, thigh, hip, pelvis, belly, chest, back, shoulders, neck, head. Breathe into the regions that are hurting and then breathe out, paying attention to the sensations you experience. Then move on.
9. For people in chronic pain, the mind tends to move to the most troublesome areas, skipping the toes and calves and hips to move, say, to the lower back or the head. That's fine. Imagine that you are breathing into the painful areas, deep into the muscles and tissues, and notice how your pain might change from moment to moment as you keep breathing in and out. If the pain subsides, try to bring your attention back to your toes and on up through your entire body.

I encourage you to look through the Resources section for more information on this powerful exercise in acceptance and present-moment awareness. Although the body scan is usually done lying down and can last for as long as an hour, if you can't just lie down on the floor because you're at work or in a public place (such as a doctor's office), do the body scan in a seated position. Even if you have just a few minutes, this technique can prove amazingly helpful. If you have several free minutes right now, turn on your computer, and try the short Body Scan Meditation offered by UCLA's Mindful Awareness Research Center (marc.ucla.edu; search for "free guided meditations"). You might want to try the other mindfulness meditations offered on this website, which range from three to nineteen minutes.

Walking Meditation

Slow down your pace of walking and focus on each movement of your legs and feet, repeating action words, such as *raising* or *moving*, in your mind and settling as you lift your foot, move your leg forward, and gently place your foot on the ground. Try to remove all thoughts of your destination, at least for a few moments. If you have pain as you walk, notice the sensations you are feeling, the actual *physical* experiences. Don't add any information about what the sensations mean; just feel them. Again, do your best to pay attention only to the physical experience, without judging what it signifies.

It may be difficult for you to stay with the physical, because you're used to interpreting what these sensations *mean*. "I can feel my disk rubbing on the nerve root," Arthur told me. "I can feel the screws moving in my spine," Gail said with a deep moan of pain. And Bill was convinced that his spine was degenerating "right now as we're sitting here in your office." Resisting the tendency to imagine what the pain means will allow you to focus on your body—either your legs and feet as they move, or your breath moving in and out of your lungs, or the specific part of your body that hurts.

"Hmmm, my back is sore," you might think, "but if I favor my right foot for a few steps, the soreness subsides." Or "I have a strong pulling sensation in my back—what happens with the next step, does it feel the same or different?" As you closely observe what happens in your body, reserving judgment about the pain's meaning or consequence, you will simply continue along. There's nothing to do, really, but walk, and breathe.

Eating Meditation

Hold in your hand a raisin, slice of apple, an almond, a carrot, or any other kind of nutritious food and spend a few minutes focusing on its texture and appearance. Then chew slowly, concentrating on your breathing, as you appreciate the nourishment that is entering your body. In her book *Help Thanks Wow*, Anne Lamott describes in exquisite detail a planned trip to the 7-Eleven to "mindlessly" buy a Hershey bar with almonds. Out of the blue, a childhood memory of eating blackberries hit her full force and she changed her mind and walked across the street to the health food store to buy a basket of blackberries:

> You eat one berry slowly, savoring the sweetness and slight resistance, and after sucking the purple juice off your fingers you say: Wow. That tasted like a very hot summer afternoon when I was about seven and walked barefoot down the dirt road to pick them off the wild blackberry bushes . . . Wow. The blackberries tasted like sweet purple nectar, not dusty exactly, but dusted just right, not quite leafy but still alive, a little bitter around the seed, juicy and warm with sunshine.

If you've ever tried to eat "mindfully," you know how challenging it can be. Arlene, 48, a nurse, described an exercise she had done that involved holding a raisin in her hand, observing its folds and valleys and noticing how light and insubstantial it felt in her hand. After a while, as instructed, she put the raisin in her mouth, chewing slowly, savoring the taste and texture, taking her time to appreciate just this one tiny raisin. She told me that she found this very difficult, since her nature is to gulp down one raisin so she can immediately put another raisin (or three or five) in her mouth, often swallowing quickly before allowing herself to truly taste them. But in one group exercise, she recounted that she was able to savor a raisin for one or two minutes, and when she really allowed herself to get into the experience, she was amazed.

"Time sort of stood still," she said, "and there was just me and the sweet juiciness of the raisin as it dissolved in my mouth, little by little. Nothing else."

Lying-Down Meditation
(Shavasana or Savasana)

In yoga, Shavasana is also called "the Corpse Pose" and it is usually practiced at the end of a yoga class. "Shavasana is an amazing tool for people in chronic pain," yoga teacher Cheryl Slader explains, "as you learn to make the conscious decision to stop identifying with your pain and all of the thoughts and stories associated with it. Shavasana will help you learn to live in the present moment, practice acceptance, and focus on positive ways to enjoy your life despite the pain."

SHAVASANA

1. Prepare for Shavasana by sitting on a mat or carpet on the floor with your knees bent, feet on the floor. Lean back onto your forearms, lift your pelvis slightly off the floor, and, with your hands, gently push the back of your pelvis toward your tailbone before returning your pelvis to the floor.
2. If you like, you can place a small pillow or cushion under your head to support the natural arch of your neck.
3. Inhale and slowly extend your right leg, then your left leg, making sure your legs are angled evenly, about 12 to 18 inches apart, to the point where your hip joints relax.
4. If you feel any discomfort, adjust your lower back, head, and neck. For people with lower back pain, bending your knees and placing your feet on the floor can help relieve any discomfort you might feel. A bolster, pillow, or folded blanket under your knees may also help relieve lower back pain.
5. Place your arms to the side, 8 to 10 inches from your body, with the palms face up.
6. Close your eyes and turn your head from one side to the other, then settle your head in the center, resting comfortably on the cushion under your neck.

7. Inhale through your nose and bring your awareness to your lungs as they expand with the breath. Notice that your belly rises with the inhalation. Without pausing, begin the exhale, continuing to breathe through your nose and allowing your abdomen to fall naturally as the air leaves your lungs. As inhalation and exhalation flow effortlessly into one another, the rhythmic nature of your breathing will be deeply relaxing.

8. If you find it difficult to still your mind ("My mind is always racing, I'm always thinking of something to do or making plans for the future," patients often say), focus on your breath, taking longer and deeper inhalations. If a thought comes up, witness the thought and allow it to pass, making space in between your thoughts and finding peace within that space.

9. Images from nature often help clear your mind of distracting thoughts. You might imagine taking a soft, feathery brush or broom and sweeping your thoughts away to the side, creating a clean and open space in your mind. Images from nature—a tranquil lake, waves gently breaking on the shore, the sun setting on distant hills—often help clear the mind of distracting thoughts.

10. As your muscles relax, your brain will calm down and distracting or stressful thoughts will begin to fall away. If thoughts continue to intrude, focus again on the slow, rhythmic inhalations and exhalations. Some people find it helpful to link a word, such as *peace* or *calm*, to the inhale and *grace* or *light* to the exhale. Find a word or phrase that is calming for you.

11. Rest in Shavasana for at least five or ten minutes, and longer if you want, but try not to fall asleep. Shavasana is said to be more relaxing than sleep because in the various stages of sleep, the mind can be very active. Just five or ten minutes of Shavasana may have the equivalent benefit of a few hours of deep sleep.

12. To exit, gently roll onto one side (preferably your right, which reduces pressure on your heart by allowing it to "rest" on top of your other organs) and exhale slowly. Take two or three breaths and on exhalation, press your hands against the floor and lift your torso, allowing your head to come up last.

13. You can end Shavasana in a seated position with the traditional practice of placing your palms together in a prayer position, taking

several deep, calming breaths. Bow to yourself and to the world outside you and say, "Namaste," a traditional Sanskrit greeting (and farewell) that means, roughly, "The Spirit within me salutes the Spirit in you."

Finding emotional equilibrium through breathing exercises, meditation, and mindfulness is a prelude (and companion) to discovering a spiritual way of life. In the next chapter we will explore together the concept of spirituality and how people living with chronic pain have found peace and serenity in simple but powerful spiritual practices.

EIGHT

REVIVING THE SPIRIT

Finding Meaning and Purpose in Your Life

The world breaks everyone and afterwards
many are strong at the broken places.

—ERNEST HEMINGWAY

So many people with chronic pain are totally consumed with their pain. All our energies are turned inward, not in a healing way but, rather, as part of a downward spiral. Our lives shrink and as the years wear on we find that we are left with little or no joy, cut off from others and from our own hearts and souls.

One of the key dynamic factors underlying both chronic pain and addiction is *self-centered fear*. For both conditions, regaining spiritual balance begins—and blossoms—with focusing on *anything other than ME!* I've heard in AA: "I'm not much, but I'm all I think about!" As we begin to turn our attention outward—toward other people, sights and colors (blue sky, green trees, crimson sunsets), sounds (music, birds singing, rhythmic breathing), and experiences (laughter, a good cry, a sense of connectedness with friends, family, and the world itself)—our consciousness gradually expands and we (our pain, our problems, our self-centered focus) become less important. Most astonishing of all, our fears and anxieties begin to dissipate as our perspective enlarges beyond our own needs and concerns.

Spirituality—finding meaning and purpose in your life—is essential for true recovery. You will need to begin to turn outward, away

185

from the darkness, toward the light, letting the sun shine on you by connecting with others who can help lighten your load. Without this outward focus—this turning away from the negative emotions you feel inside to explore and discover the peace, serenity, and joy of loving relationships—healing cannot take place.

How can you find strength in the broken places? In this chapter, I am not going to offer you seven simple strategies, ten trendy tips, or eight easy steps to a spiritual life. You know enough about life, pain, and loss to reject a Band-Aid stretched across a gaping wound. Instead, this chapter explores how a spiritual way of living is an antidote to the suffering associated with chronic pain. These insights and strategies will help you transcend your pain and discover new meaning in life.

WHAT IS SPIRITUALITY?

The first and most important thing to remember about spirituality is that it is not easy to define. Recently I was reminded of this in the pain group I facilitate every Tuesday at one p.m. Participating in this group is my favorite activity of the week, giving me the opportunity to sit and visit with all the patients in the pain program (usually six to twelve people at one time). They are in various stages of healing—some have just arrived, others have been in the program for a few weeks or more, and there are usually a few patients nearing the end of their stay in treatment who add their wisdom and experience, more often than not reporting low pain levels and new insights into their lives, their pasts, and their plans for what comes next.

Something happens as people share their stories—their wisdom, strength, and hope—and those who listen understand, often for the first time, that they are not alone. What I witness is as close to a miracle as I've ever seen.

On this particular day I asked a group of eight patients, several of whom were also struggling with addiction to opioids, "What is spirituality?" The answers came slowly, at first, but eventually everyone in the group offered their thoughts and several kept adding to the list. *Faith. Freedom. Peace. Meditation. Acceptance. Acceptance of who I am. Higher Power* (God, Buddha, Jesus, Allah, . . .). *Trust. Vulnerability. Honesty. Hope. Being less self-centered. Compassion. Connection with others.*

Each person has his or her own way of defining spirituality because, in many senses, spirituality is impossible to define. It can only be experienced. And like chronic pain, it is universal, yet uniquely different for each and every one of us. As different as we may be, however, one spiritual truth is universal and constant—we need one another.

Developing relationships that are supportive and nurturing is a critically important element of pain recovery. You need to feel understood and to find people with whom you can identify. Mutual aid or self-help support groups are invaluable, for in those groups—in the rooms, around the tables—you will find friends and allies who understand pain, in all its multifaceted complexity. When you attend a support group for people in chronic pain, you will discover that you are not alone. That discovery, in and of itself, can be life-changing. I find that the underlying spiritual principles of the Twelve Steps work just as well for people living with chronic pain as they do for people living with addiction.

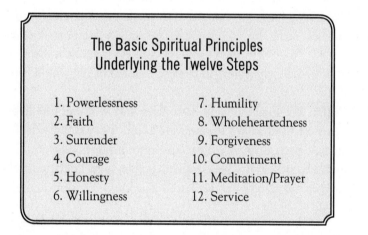

The Basic Spiritual Principles Underlying the Twelve Steps

1. Powerlessness
2. Faith
3. Surrender
4. Courage
5. Honesty
6. Willingness
7. Humility
8. Wholeheartedness
9. Forgiveness
10. Commitment
11. Meditation/Prayer
12. Service

In 2006, soon after the establishment of LVRC's pain recovery program, I met with a group of colleagues at the center to create a support group based on the Twelve Steps, but specifically for people for whom medication-based approaches have not worked and who need support for abstinence-based pain relief and recovery. While PIRSG (Pain in Recovery Support Group) embraces the principles of the Twelve Steps, these groups are not intended to be a substitute for involvement in Twelve-Step fellowships, only to complement them. Here are the

Twelve Steps with suggestions on how to use them in your recovery from chronic pain.

STEP ONE: We admitted we were powerless over our chronic pain, and that our lives had become unmanageable. The first step with chronic pain, as with addiction, is to surrender control by admitting that we are powerless over having chronic pain and it has created unmanageability in our lives. Accepting that we are powerless over chronic pain allows us to stop investing time, emotion, and energy into fighting against and resisting it. Our reactions to chronic pain only increased our suffering and unmanageability.

STEP TWO: We came to believe that a power greater than ourselves could restore us to sanity. In the second step, we begin to see how the unmanageability of our chronic pain contributes to various forms of insanity and irrationality in our lives, such as obsessing on our pain and suffering, taking more pain medication while receiving less actual pain relief, and excusing our use of opioids because a doctor said we needed to take them. We begin the process of connecting with a power greater than ourselves to help restore us to sane/rational thinking and behaving.

STEP THREE: We made a decision to turn our will and our lives over to the care of God as we understood Him. By making a decision to turn our will and our lives over to the care of our higher power in the third step, we consciously seek out this higher-level guidance and use it to support healthy, recovery-oriented thinking, decision-making, and actions.

STEP FOUR: We made a searching and fearless moral inventory of ourselves. In the fourth step, we make a thorough and courageous inventory of ourselves related to chronic pain. We take a close and careful look at our resentments, fears, shame and guilt, relationships, and other important life areas that have been affected as a result of living with chronic pain. Through this process, we can get a clear picture of how pain has impacted our lives and the lives of others.

STEP FIVE: We admitted to God, to ourselves, and to another human being the exact nature of our wrongs. We gain clarity in the fifth step by admitting the exact nature of our wrongdoings, in addition to our suffering, to our higher power, ourselves, and another person. In recovery from pain, as well as addiction, danger lies in keeping secrets and self-deceptions hidden and in not sharing them. When such things are spoken, they become less threatening, less overwhelming, and much clearer.

STEP SIX: **We were entirely ready to have God remove these defects of character.** In the sixth step, we identify the aspects or defects of our character that form the foundation of the exact nature of our wrong-doings. These defects are basic challenging personality traits that are common to most people, but have created more serious problems in our lives and the lives of those closest to us due to the self-centeredness that goes hand-in-hand with both chronic pain and addiction. We assess how these character traits manifest themselves in our lives and become ready to let go of them.

STEP SEVEN: **We humbly asked Him to remove our shortcomings.** The seventh step provides us with the opportunity to connect specific behaviors or shortcomings with our character challenges. We identify the spiritual principles that represent the opposites of our defects, for example, acceptance, trust, responsibility, humility, gratitude, patience, compassion, and positive action and begin to practice these principles in our lives. We draw on our relationship with a power greater than ourselves in working to shed old, self-defeating ways of thinking and acting.

STEP EIGHT: **We made a list of all persons we had harmed, and became willing to make amends to them all.** As a result of the ways in which we acted out on our character defects and sufferings, in response to our pain, we harmed others. In the eighth step, we identify who we have wronged and how we wronged them. In our pain and self-centered fear we may have justified the wrongdoings we did to others as an unavoidable consequence of our pain. We became ready to do what we can to repair the damage we have caused and willing to make amends to those we have harmed.

STEP NINE: **We made direct amends to such people wherever possible, except when to do so would injure them or others.** In making such amends we find the capacity to forgive ourselves and accept forgiveness from others when it is offered. Even in the instances when we are not forgiven, we still find freedom from the past.

STEP TEN: We continued to take personal inventory, and when we were wrong, promptly admitted it. By taking a daily personal inventory in the tenth step, we strengthen our ability to stay in the moment and live with chronic pain one day at a time. We strive to become consciously aware of our thoughts and actions in an ongoing way. We try to maintain nonjudgmental mindfulness with regard to how we relate to ourselves, to others, and to the world. Whenever we become aware that we have committed some wrongdoing, we admit this and take responsibility for it.

STEP ELEVEN: We sought through prayer and meditation to increase our conscious contact with God as we understood Him, praying only for the knowledge of His will for us and the power to carry it out. The eleventh step emphasizes the healing value of an ongoing relationship with a power greater than ourselves; the higher power of our own choosing that has helped restore us to sanity.

STEP TWELVE: Having had a spiritual awakening as the result of these steps, we tried to carry this message to others who suffer from chronic pain, and to practice these principles in all our affairs. In the twelfth step, we continue applying the principles we have learned in each of the proceeding steps and carry the message of pain recovery to others. The spiritual awakening referred to in this step does not have to be dramatic or earth-shaking; in fact, it can consist of the simple realization that by accepting life on its own terms, including our chronic pain, we can experience much more contentment and serenity than we ever could by continuing to oppose, resist, and fight against it. One of the universal truths of recovery is that we can keep what we have most effectively by giving it away.

Many people in Twelve Step programs view "God" as an acronym for "Group of Drunks" or "Good Orderly Direction." You can substitute Allah, Hashem, Jah, Yahweh, Universal Life Force, the Divine, World Spirit, Nature, or any variation that makes sense to you and brings you comfort. Buddhism is a non-theistic religion, which means that God is not part of the discussion, although, for me, a higher power or force (I'm okay with calling it "God") is part of my belief system, and I also resonate with Buddhist ideology that tells us that God is embodied in each of us. The point is that your unique and individual spiritual beliefs allow you to choose whatever Higher Power you want.

If you do not find what you are looking for in religion or the Twelve Steps, there are many other spiritual pathways available to you. The Dalai Lama reminds us that the basic philosophy underlying all religions and spiritual traditions is kindness toward ourselves and others:

> This is my simple religion. There is no need for temples; no need for complicated philosophy. Our own brain, our own heart is our temple; the philosophy is kindness.

Something Helpless That Needs Our Help

The Twelve Steps—in whatever form they appear and however you are willing to accept them—do not lead to a higher, more elevated spiritual state. Instead, they ground us in "what is" and allow us to find a place of balance within the awareness and acceptance of the everyday challenges of our lives. Living with chronic pain, whether or not drugs are involved, can be a daily struggle to find a place of balance. Spiritual balance is especially tricky, because it is so difficult to pin down—for again, what is spirituality? Specifically, what role does spirituality have in understanding and dealing with chronic pain? A favorite quotation may offer some insights:

> Everything terrifying is, in its deepest being, something helpless that needs our help.

When I first read this quotation by Bohemian-Austrian poet Rainer Maria Rilke I focused on the word *terrifying* and asked myself, "Isn't *terror* exaggerating a bit?" On reflection, however, I know that I have felt terror when confronting my pain. Those nights when I'd wake up and be unable to go back to sleep because of the pain, I'd think, "This is worse than ever, it's going to be like this forever." Or those days when

I'd be working with a chronic pain patient and have to grit my teeth to get through the session because my low back was aching and throbbing. Yes, sure, at times I felt terrified.

The more I thought about the quote, the more meaningful it became. Using Rilke's imagery, thinking of my pain as "helpless" changed things for me. The pain wasn't my enemy, nor was it something I could eliminate, cut out, burn away, or dissolve. Believe me, I have tried, but no matter what I did over the years, the pain was still there. It will always be there to some degree or other. But that is not to say that it "wants" to be there, that it "wants" to torment me, that it "wants" to take over and control my life.

Dustin had seven back surgeries. His pain levels were always high, regardless of what medications he took. If he took a handful of Percocet with a few Soma and an Ambien, he could doze in his chair and get an hour's relief. "I hate my life and this f-ing pain," he said, near tears. "It's a curse, God's punishment for being a bad guy. This pain wants me to be miserable and it has taken over my life!"

Chronic pain doesn't "want" anything. The pain is just there, and so the only choice, really, is to accept it and learn to peacefully coexist with it. This reminds me of a Randall Jarrell quote: "Pain comes from the darkness. And we call it wisdom. It is pain." Of course you can refuse to accept pain, try to get away from it, and tighten against it, which is the primary coping style I see in most patients I work with—armor up, resist, attempt to twist away. But the pain always gets worse when you turn away from it. Rilke's words urge you to recognize and acknowledge that you are more powerful than your pain, and *it needs your help*.

What kind of help can you offer your pain? You can pay attention to it, be aware of it, get to know it, become more comfortable with it being a part of you, soothe it, and comfort it. I know, this might sound a little crazy—but ignoring the pain or pretending it doesn't exist, wishing it away, loathing it, and fighting it hasn't worked for me or countless patients I have treated. We only end up hating it more, and when and if it gets worse, we hate ourselves more.

That realization—hating your pain means hating yourself—may give you a glimpse of freedom. You can live with pain and, at the same time, be free from pain's terrifying presence. You don't want to spend your time hating your back, your pain, yourself. You don't want to spend even a moment being mean to yourself. If your pain is part of you, if it isn't malicious or evil, if it is just some crossed wires deep in the marvelously intricate neurocircuitry of your brain, above and beyond your conscious control, then it does you no good to put so much negative energy into it. So, when your pain flares up, try to think about how those tender, sore places need your help rather than your antipathy. Your body is sending you messages. "Slow down, pay attention! Where are your thoughts taking you? What is bothering you? What memories are disturbing or upsetting you? What can you do to feel better?" Try to respond to these messages with awareness, tenderness, and compassion.

I encourage you to reread the last few pages, reflect, and write about these concepts. What realizations or insights do you have? How can you treat your body with more tender, loving care? How is your pain helpless and why does it need your help? What can you do to be kinder toward yourself and less terrified of your pain? These questions will help ground you, and once you are released from the intensity of the emotions connected to your pain, you can move toward gratitude.

GRATITUDE

The following story, adapted from a May 10, 2014, *New York Times* article titled "A Soldier's War on Pain," is a great illustration of the healing power of gratitude.

Sergeant Shane Savage was seriously injured when a roadside bomb blew apart the armored truck he was commanding near Kandahar, Afghanistan. His foot was pinned against the truck's dashboard, crushing twenty-four bones, and his head hit the roof so hard that his helmet cracked. Back at Fort Hood in Killeen, Texas, doctors diagnosed Sergeant Savage as having post-traumatic stress and chronic pain. The doctors prescribed a bunch of drugs—including opioids. The pain didn't let up, nor did the dosages—after numerous surgeries to repair his shattered foot, he was taking over 300 milligrams of morphine per day, which is three times the dose considered safe by experts in pain treatment.

When Sergeant Savage enrolled in a pain program at the Veterans Affairs Medical Center in San Francisco, he received the help he needed to get off all narcotic drugs. After many more surgeries that failed to reconstruct his foot, he is now preparing for an amputation of part of his left leg, from the middle of his calf down. He will wear a prosthetic device.

"You have to find alternative ways to get out and do stuff to stay active, to get your brain off the thought process of 'I'm in pain,'" Sergeant Savage told *New York Times* reporter Barry Meier. "Am I the person that I was four years ago? No. Will I ever be? No. Will I ever be able to run down the street and chase my girls? I really don't know," he said. "But you know what? I can get a bike and I can ride with them."

■ ■ ■

An older, almost timeless story about "something missing" always chokes me up. I first read this story in Kathy's book *The Spirituality of Imperfection*, coauthored by Ernest Kurtz. Every time I read it, I am reminded to be grateful for all that I have, for all the parts and pieces of my life that I too often take for granted.

■   A blind man was begging in a city park. Someone approached and asked him whether people were giving generously. The blind man shook a nearly empty tin.

His visitor said to him, "Let me write something on your card." The blind man agreed. That evening the visitor returned. "Well, how were things today?"

The blind man showed him a tin full of money and asked, "What on earth did you write on that card?"

"Oh," said the other, "I merely wrote 'Today is a spring day, and I am blind.'"

■ ■ ■

Keep a Gratitude Journal

What are you grateful for? So much has been taken from you, but so much remains that is of value—even priceless. I recommend that you keep a Gratitude Journal, at least for a while, to remind you of all the good in your life. It's simple. You can use an inexpensive note pad, a lined or unlined journal from a stationery store, or a yellow legal pad, which is where much of my journaling ends up. Every night or morning, write down five things for which you are grateful. Try to write in your journal every day, but don't beat yourself up if you forget for a day or a week. It's fine if you repeat yourself—no rules here—but chances are that this spiritual practice will lead you toward peace and appreciation for what is good in your life.

Not everyone enjoys writing in a journal. Sometimes just listing the gifts in your life—and adding to that list whenever you want—fosters the experience of gratitude. Kathleen was forty years old when she went to the doctor for fatigue, exhaustion, achy and painful joints, insomnia, and what she called "brain fog." After multiple tests, diagnoses, and visits to specialists, she was diagnosed with palindromic arthritis, a rare type of inflammatory arthritis involving sudden and acute attacks in several joints. She manages the recurrent flare-ups with ibuprofen and a gluten- and dairy-free diet.

A few weeks after her fiftieth birthday Kathleen created this gratitude list.

I'm grateful:
for a loving husband,
that my daughters are married to good men, and all live nearby,
that I get to spend lots of time with my grandkids, reading, swinging, walking, and hugging,
for financial stability,
for our country home along the river,
for morning walks along the river with a hot cup of coffee,
for sunrises & sunsets,
that I get to be lulled to sleep by crickets, frogs, and the roar of the river,
for living with horses, alpacas, dogs, and cats, who remind me to live in the moment,
for being able to bury my face in my horses manes and inhale,
for riding my horse in the local parades with friends,
for rainbows after a good storm,
for wine & laughter with friends,
for fresh tomatoes and cucumbers from my small garden,
for having wild apple trees, plum trees, & blackberry bushes on our property,
for canned applesauce and blackberry jam to enjoy through the winter months,

for the many projects on our property that keep me and my husband physically active,

for quiet moments lounging on my back porch listening to the sounds of nature,

for being aware that lounging is okay . . .

Whenever I look at a list like Kathleen's, I think of my old friend George, who used to thank his higher power "all through the day" for the "goodies" he had in his daily life. Although he died over ten years ago, many of us in my AA group lovingly remember George's words as we find ourselves appreciating the little things we have all through the day—a cool breeze on a hot day, a good laugh, a few minutes without pain. Do you have a gratitude list? The following template may help you "count your blessings." Use the blank spaces to describe what you are grateful for and why.

I Am Grateful For:	Because . . .
My family	
My friends	
My children	
My partner	
The kind of friend I am	
The kind of parent I am	
The kind of person I am	
My body	
My values and character	
My intelligence	
My intuition	
My talents	
My hobbies	
My willingness to change	
My compassion	

ACCEPTANCE

When we discover gratitude for what we have and focus on "gifts" rather than "losses," a dawning acceptance often takes place.

"I will not accept this misery as my life sentence!" Suzanna glared at me defiantly.

"Okay," I responded. "Tell me, then, what choices do you have? You've told me you can't use pain pills any longer because they caused you so many problems, and another surgery is definitely out, so what's left?"

She began to sob, and I sat silently with her. I felt helpless. After all, I was unable to change the fact that she had titanium rods in her back or the progressive arthritis that afflicted her. I could only tell her the truth—I believed she had only one route to take. Acceptance.

When she looked up, something had changed. The tension around her mouth was gone, the glare was softened. She looked me in the eyes and much to my surprise and joy she said, simply, "Okay, let's do this." And she began to get better.

When Suzanna stopped living and breathing in the depths of her suffering, her sense of helplessness and hopelessness began to dissipate. She stopped fighting the reality of her life and made a commitment to invest her time and energy in the difficult but rewarding work of recovery. In a word, she surrendered, accepting her pain, and from that point on she was able to focus on learning how to live with it.

The Serenity Prayer is all about acceptance. While it's called a prayer, it can just as easily be a meditation or an exercise in gratitude. As for the "God" word—I know many atheists and agnostics who find great peace and joy in this prayer but who leave out the first word or substitute the "God" of their understanding. Here is the original version of the first two verses of the Serenity Prayer by theologian Reinhold Niebuhr.

The Serenity Prayer
By Reinhold Niebuhr

God, give me grace to accept with serenity
the things that cannot be changed,

Courage to change the things
which should be changed,
and the Wisdom to distinguish
the one from the other.

Living one day at a time,
Enjoying one moment at a time,
Accepting hardship as a pathway to peace . . .

GRIEVING FOR WHAT WE HAVE LOST

Grieving for what we have lost is a natural and necessary process that we all go through and which can often last for years. Because life consists of many losses, you may go through the multistage grief process several times. You may have heard of the Kübler-Ross model of the Five Stages of Grief, which is applicable here. First comes Denial, in which we try to wall ourselves off from the grim reality of our situation by creating a false reality.

Tommy was clearly in denial in pain group. His pain levels were unrelentingly high, and he was sure the program was not for him. All he needed, he insisted, was to be back on his pain medications but at higher levels than he'd previously taken. Despite the fact that he had totaled his car the week before he arrived, he told the group: "My life was fine before I got here—my wife and kids got all upset after one incident when I took too many pills and blew it completely out of proportion."

Next comes Anger as the pain continues and the truth begins to sink in. This is the "Why me? It's just not fair!" stage.

"Yeah, everyone just overreacted," Tommy said, "and so I'm here, suffering needlessly. I want to put my fist through the wall. I have half a mind to just leave my damn family once and for all."

The third stage of grief is Bargaining. I'll never forget Lindsay, a forty-two-year-old school bus driver who tried bargaining with me. "Okay, Doc, no more pills unless I really need one, right? I was using twenty or thirty pills a day—I want to cut down to five or six like I used to take, just to take the edge off my pain. Okay?" My answer didn't please her. "No, Lindsay, not okay," I said. "For you, taking one pill turns into twenty or more. Your brain needs to be off opioids for a few weeks and then you will start to hurt less. Taking just one pill will start the dependence all over again."

The fourth stage is Depression. For many if not most people living with chronic pain, this is the "stuck" stage when they ask themselves, "What's the point? Why bother? Nobody understands. People are tired of me. I'm tired of me! My doctors can't stand to see me. My friends are abandoning me. I'm never going to feel any better, and this pain is never going away." This stage is totally self-involved for it is all about feeling sorry for yourself.

When Lindsay heard my explanation, she got a flat, sad, hopeless look on her face. "I can't go on without the pills, Doc! I just can't live without them. I don't want to lose my family or my job, you've got to believe me, but I'm so miserable without the pills. I'd be better off dead."

Oddly enough, these are the thoughts and feelings that lead to the final, fifth step in the grief process: Acceptance. Sergio had come a long way, shifting his attitude from bitter, resentful, distant, and un-approachable to a calm composure and sense of peacefulness that affected everyone in group. His attitude had changed dramatically in the week since we had last met. "Doc," he said with a big smile, "when I stopped fighting with you and everyone else, the problems seemed to shrink, my shoulders relaxed, and I stopped hurting so much. I guess that's the acceptance I've heard everyone talk about so much. I sure like it better this way!"

Science confirms that the ability to "accept the things I cannot change" helps people with chronic pain (and addictions) live in the moment rather than catastrophize about the future. Through the acceptance of pain and other "unwanted" experiences, we disarm our fear and depression. In a 2014 article titled "Mindfulness, Acceptance and Catastrophizing in Chronic Pain," researchers conclude that an accepting attitude "may prevent a person with pain from catastrophizing and may . . . prevent the development of fear of pain, avoidance, hypervigilance, disuse, depression and disability."

JODY'S STORY

Fifteen years ago, when I was in my early forties, I was diagnosed with Lyme disease. I started getting numbness around my lips and weird sensations in my legs. Back then nobody really believed in the disease and every doctor had a different theory. Now they know a lot more.

Fear can grow and grow, so when something goes wrong, I've gotten really good at going straight to the doctor. I accept what is and try to make the experience as positive as I can.

When I have flare-ups, it's important to manage my stress levels. Rather than letting things percolate so they grow out of control and feel scarier (when they might not be anything), I go toward them—acknowledging and accepting, making the best of it.

My life has been filled with a string of tragedies dating back to my childhood. My father was killed in a car accident when I was a teenager, a precious friend committed suicide, one daughter died soon after being born, my beloved husband lost a battle with cancer, and my extraordinary second daughter died more recently from a rare degenerative disorder.

Of course, I never imagined that life would hand me any of these circumstances, but unfortunately, I wasn't consulted. The reality is we don't get a memo when bad things are about to happen. Life just smacks us upside the head and we have to find a way to bear the unbearable. That's our choice—sink or swim—or at the very least . . . learn to float, going with the current, not fighting it.

A few years ago, two friends invited me to a workshop at the Open Center in NYC. The author Thomas Moore, whose book *Dark Nights of the Soul* had just been released, was presenting. As the seminar came to a close, my friends urged me to talk to him. I resisted, but they were concerned about me and persevered.

"Perhaps he'll have some useful input on your situation," they said.

After the room had cleared and it felt a bit more private, I approached this gentle, tall man with a kind voice. I was surprised when a lump began to form in my throat as I considered what to say. Unprepared, I whispered, "Do you have any advice for a person whose life seems to be filled with one tragedy after another?" I found myself fighting back tears. Even so, he looked me straight in the eyes and firmly said,

"Yes, I do." (Followed by a very long pause.) "That's your life, accept it."

Our eyes stayed linked as I shook my head in agreement. Although unexpected, at the very moment he said it, Thomas Moore's response "rang true" to me. Not exactly "suck it up," but certainly a close relative.

Sometimes, when disaster strikes, sinking feels like the easiest choice for it allows us to disappear. Often unprepared, we struggle to process what's happened and simply go down. It's natural to think that the alternative to sinking involves action as we struggle to do anything to improve a situation. But the reality is, it's often not possible to fix things and all the frantic activity simply creates a rip current, once again, removing us emotionally. "Floating," on the other hand, is different for it uses less energy. It involves going with the current, not fighting it. When you float through difficulty, the limited available energy can be channeled more effectively into the needs of the heart.

■ ■ ■

FORGIVENESS

Forgiveness is giving up all hope of having had a better past.

—ANNE LAMOTT

Acceptance of self and others leads us to another spiritual reality—forgiveness. As with gratitude and acceptance, researchers are offering actual proof that the inability to forgive is directly linked to the intensity of the pain we experience. A 2005 Duke University study shows that people with chronic lower back pain who report an inability to forgive others tend to experience higher pain levels, whereas people who report high levels of forgiveness report lower levels of pain and psychological distress. Neuropsychologists at the University of Arizona conducted studies suggesting that forgiveness alleviates lower back pain by disrupting patterns of fear and stress in the midbrain's limbic system or "the emotional" brain, which in turn reduces the level of circulating stress hormones and eases muscle tension. The theory is that forgiveness stops the midbrain from storing away new memories of pain and distress and helps the brain create new memories that encourage the process of long-term pain recovery.

The narratives we tell ourselves become part of who we are and how we react and interact with others. If you consistently feel offended or tormented by the words or actions of others, blaming the "offender" for the pain and psychological distress that you feel, you are unconsciously creating grievance stories that will perpetuate and intensify your physical and emotional misery. How freeing it is to let go of those old, useless, self-destructive feelings by practicing forgiveness! And how relatively painless, compared to the alternatives. As Martin Luther King, Jr. explained: "Darkness cannot drive out darkness; only light can do that. Hate cannot drive out hate; only love can do that."

I had a significant experience in forgiving my father for imparting to me the feeling that I was never enough. He did this inadvertently and unwittingly and surely not because he didn't love me. Nevertheless, over time I developed a sense of not being adequate as I was. He once looked at my report card and said: "Only an A?" I didn't have the heart to tell him there were no A-pluses in my school, and so I just internalized one more time a sense of falling short of his standards. That memory challenges me to this day. I am certain he meant only the best for me for he was a good and loving father, but there was so much that I wanted about him to be different.

Many years ago at an AA meeting, a man about my age was talking about his father. "He did the best he could with what he had," he said. When I heard those words, simple and often repeated as they are, I was really moved. In that context, at that particular moment, the words struck deep, and I had trouble catching my breath. I began to cry. For the first time, I had a different sense of my father, and that feeling of sudden, unbidden forgiveness has sustained me ever since.

"She did the best with what she could." I use this line with patients all the time, and for many, it strikes home as it did for me. I recently received a note from a former patient who told me that these words had a profound impact on her, allowing her to forgive her abusive, neglectful mother and, in the process, she discovered forgiveness for herself.

But how does one "practice" forgiveness? How do you forgive? I strongly recommend that you listen to Jack Kornfield's powerful meditations on forgiveness and self-forgiveness (see the Resources section). Here is one of his meditations I practice and introduce to patients during group from time to time.

There are many ways that I have hurt and harmed myself. I have betrayed or abandoned myself many times through thought, word, or deed, knowingly or unknowingly. Feel your own precious body and life. Let yourself see the ways you have hurt or harmed yourself.

Picture them, remember them. Feel the sorrow you have carried from this and sense that you can release these burdens. Extend forgiveness for each of them, one by one. Repeat to yourself: For the ways I have hurt myself through action or inaction, out of fear, pain and confusion, I now extend a full and heartfelt forgiveness. I forgive myself, I forgive myself.

The meditation goes on to instruct you to forgive those who hurt or harmed you and ask forgiveness for those whom you have hurt or harmed.

The word *give* in *forgiveness* is part of its deep power. Giving up attachment to a sense of woundedness—that feeling of victimhood—is an important and, I would add, essential step in the process of forgiveness. Giving up the hope that we can somehow change the past is a different way of saying the same thing. Consciously, if slowly and even somewhat painfully, we break the chains to the past and the scars that cannot heal because we continue to rip them open in our minds and our memories.

Letting go of past hurts is difficult work in large part because it involves forgiveness of one's own self. As a team of Seattle University scholars explain in a paper titled "The Psychology of Forgiving Another":

> An important aspect of the self-forgiveness process is experiencing the grief that comes with letting go—grieving for what might have been, feeling regret for what was, accepting who one is . . .
>
> One also comes to a new understanding of responsibility. Where before one was primarily in a denying or blaming stance toward self, now there is the honest acknowledgement of participation in the event. This awareness of responsibility frees one to move into a more accepting relationship with self. Thus, self-forgiveness involves a shift from estrangement to being at home with one's self and others. It involves accepting one's own humanness.

I think the practice of forgiveness begins right there—not with forgiving others, but with forgiving ourselves. And in forgiving ourselves, the doors to forgiving others are flung wide open.

Forgiveness is something we all seek, in some ways, as this oft-told story so poignantly illustrates. (The original version appeared in Ernest Hemingway's short story "The Capital of the World.")

A father and his son were estranged. The son, whose name was Paco, had wronged his father and in his shame, he had run away from home. The father searched all over Spain to find his son, but to no avail. Finally, in a last desperate attempt, he placed an ad in a Madrid newspaper. "Dear Paco," the ad read, "please meet me at the Hotel Montana. Tuesday at noon. All is forgiven. I love you. Your father."

On Tuesday 800 Pacos showed up, looking for forgiveness and love from their fathers.

LISTENING

The best "healing" work I can do with my patients is to listen. I'm amazed at the change that takes place when patients spend some time with me—not because I've said something cosmic or worked some medical miracle, but because they have been allowed to express themselves, cry, laugh, shout, and share intimate details of their tough life experiences with an interested, empathic listener. This is the essence of making a spiritual connection.

Often it is not the words that my patients say, but what they don't say that tells me what I need to know. I "listen" to Tina's pain by noticing the way she leans forward in her chair, as if folding over to protect herself. I "listen" to Marty's anger by watching his jaw tense and his eyes narrow. I "listen" to Jeff's story of sexual abuse by witnessing his tears and waiting patiently during his silences. I "listen" by offering my time, by waiting, watching, caring, and being fully, wholly present. Through my silences as much as my words, I let my patients know that I am in no hurry, that I will stay with them, be with them, care for them.

To emphasize the importance of sensitive, empathic listening, I like to use a "listening exercise" in my sessions with patients and also in our family sessions. I pair up two people and ask one person to talk about whatever topic is introduced, while the other is simply to stay quiet, attentive, nodding but not asking questions or sharing his or her own experiences. "Just listen," I instruct, "mouth closed." After five or ten minutes, they switch roles, so that each has the experience of listening and being listened to. Try this simple exercise with a friend or spouse, and you'll be amazed at how good it feels to have someone listen, truly listen without interruption—and what a gift it can be to another person to listen attentively without saying a word.

We all need people in our lives who listen to us with compassion and empathy, and we also need to learn how to be good listeners ourselves. Jim, diagnosed with multiple sclerosis at age thirty-two, learned about the importance of listening when he decided to stop taking the high doses of methadone his doctor prescribed for his chronic pain.

Anyone who has gone through hell to get clean and sober loves to talk about his or her experience. It's very cathartic to unleash everything that has built up over months and years of using even if you took drugs only as prescribed. It feels good to tell your story. And in some ways I think people are looking for affirmation that they've done well.

My wife was the only person I talked to about what I was going through. She never drank or used any type of drugs in her life. But she listened intently, witnessing my ups and downs in the first few months and taking it all in stride. She didn't have any advice, she just let me sound off, I guess. She did try to help me stay positive and reassured me that I would start to feel better soon.

Sometimes people like to vent and are not really searching for answers or advice or wanting the other person to "fix things." Just hearing the other person is enough in most cases. Looking back it seems what I went through was a lifetime ago. I do know for a fact that if my MS were to relapse I wouldn't go back on narcotics. I would take whatever I had to, but it would be non-narcotic. I never want to get to the place that I was. It zapped me physically and more importantly spiritually and made me a numbed out human being.

But I don't let what I went through define me. I don't focus on it and I stopped talking about it to my wife a long time ago. It's in the past and I can't do a thing to change that. So, I just look forward to the future and live in the present.

Here are some simple steps you can take to help you become a better listener—and to help your friends and family members learn how to listen sensitively and compassionately.

Five Steps to Empathic Listening

1. **Pay attention.** Focus in and pay attention, not just on the words being spoken but to gestures, general posture, body position, and facial expressions. Often what we don't say is as important as what we do say!

2. **Be silent.** The words *silent* and *listen* contain the same letters. This step takes lots of practice! Some people find that even a simple "Hmmm" or "uh-huh" can be annoying and distracting when they are talking. Being silent also means that the listener does not shift around in his or her chair, yawn, stretch, stare out the window, tap a pen against the chair or table, or sneak a look at a watch or cell phone.

3. **Ask questions.** Always give the speaker the opportunity to explain him- or herself fully before you respond. We all have a tendency to interrupt, offering our own perspective or biases, jumping off someone's story to tell a story of our own, or just completely switching the subject. Being aware of this tendency, make sure you ask questions and allow the person to fully reveal his or her thoughts and feelings before it is your turn to speak.

4. **Accept without judgment.** Listen without condoning or condemning, giving up the idea that you need to agree or disagree with the speaker. Avoid advising, criticizing, judging, or fixing. Know that the art of listening is all about the effort to understand what the other person is saying.

5. **Check in.** When the person is finished speaking, wait a moment and then "check in" to make sure you have "heard" what he or she is trying to say. You might say, "Just to be sure I understand, I think you might be saying . . . " or "Correct me if I'm misunderstanding you, but it seems that you might be feeling . . . "

Good listening is letting another person know that we are there, that we are paying attention, and that what that person says—and doesn't or cannot say at that moment—matters to us. Through paying attention and truly listening, we commune with one another, and we create a community. As the philosopher Hans-Georg Gadamer pointed out: "Hearing implies already belonging together in such a manner that one is claimed by what is being said."

We belong together. I believe those three words sum up the essence of our search for meaning. Because we struggle and because we sometimes fail—we need each other. Or, as Dag Hammarskjöld said,

> *What makes loneliness an anguish*
> *Is not that I have no one to share my burden,*
> *But this:*
> *I have only my own burden to bear.*

Part 3

MOVING FORWARD

Is it not time that lovingly we freed ourselves
. . . and, quivering, endured:
as the arrow endures the bow-string's tension
and in this tense release becomes more than itself.
For staying is nowhere.

—RAINER MARIA RILKE

We've covered a lot of ground in Parts 1 and 2. You might be wondering, "Where do I begin? How do I get started?"

"Staying is nowhere," as Rilke writes. In these final chapters you will find the information you need to move forward. In Chapter 9 we offer a four-week Jump Start Plan with simple, straightforward strategies to help you choose which steps to take first and from there, how to build a daily regimen that you can sustain through time. Chapter 10 offers a comprehensive overview of the impact of nutrition on pain—what you eat and drink and how you prepare your meals—along with an abundance of useful suggestions. In Chapter 11 Kathy and I leave you with a tried-and-true formula for the Pain Antidote and a final story of courage, strength, wisdom, and grace.

We wish you good work . . . and pain-free moments every day!

NINE

THE JUMP START PLAN
Keeping It Simple

Magic is believing in yourself.
If you can do that, you can make anything happen.
—JOHANN WOLFGANG VON GOETHE

"What is it you plan to do with your one wild and precious life?" asks poet Mary Gordon. That is the question we must all ask as we move forward in our healing journey. For those of us living with chronic pain, it's important to remember that we need to start slow and keep it simple. Chronic pain can be overwhelming in and of itself, and when given too many choices, you may be tempted to duck and run for cover. I often hear complaints from new patients admitted to the center:

- "I can't do everything you are asking me to do!"
- "I'm used to taking a two-hour nap and sitting in a recliner watching TV for most of the day—how do you expect me to work out with the trainer and go to groups all day and meetings at night?"
- "This is just not for me, especially yoga!"
- "There's no way I'm going to sit for twenty minutes every day and meditate!"

My first recommendation is, "Relax!" Moderation, balance, and sustainability are the keys to this process. I'd much rather you meditate five or ten minutes every day than twenty or thirty minutes for a few days, find it's too much, and quit trying. Likewise, changing one element of your diet (eliminating sugar, for example, or bread, or soda, whichever is easiest) may be achievable long term—if not, then eliminate doughnuts or bagels for a time and see how that feels.

The Jump Start Plan isn't about deprivation—it's about making your life better. Some of the measures will take discipline, though, so it's important for you to know what you're in for right from the start. And you will need to make a commitment to stick with the plan for the long term if these recommendations are going to make a real and lasting difference in your life.

An Important Note About Medications

You probably have gleaned by now that I am not a fan of opioids for the long-term treatment of chronic pain. There is little or no evidence that they work. You may disagree, from your experience—and if you are taking opioids and they are helping you have a better life, then I support your continuing to take them. Whether or not you are taking opioids, I encourage you to benefit from all of the information in this book. If you've decided that opioids are not making your life better, then, perhaps, it's time to consider decreasing or stopping them.

Opioids are potent drugs that have the potential to bind tightly to the receptors in your body. Therefore, if you want to cut down on the dose or stop, you will be facing a physical and emotional challenge your system will likely not feel good about parting with these powerful substances. There are two basic ways to approach withdrawal: One is to gradually cut down the dose, realizing that each time you decrease your dose, you are likely to get a "pain spike" related to withdrawal. These spikes are temporary because withdrawal symptoms subside over time, but with each downward dosage adjustment, you are likely to experience another pain spike.

Always consult with your prescribing physician about such a plan. Inquire whether your prescriber has experience in weaning people down to lower doses of medicine. As with detoxification, there are medications

continues

continued

that can ease the unpleasant symptoms associated with coming off these medications (for example, Clonidine for anxiety, elevated pulse and blood pressure; Robaxin or Baclofen for muscle spasms; trazadone or amitriptyline for sleep; Vistaril and/or phenobarbital for anxiety; Bentyl for stomach cramps).

If you are gradually decreasing the dose of medication under the supervision of a physician, you may find a dose associated with fewer side effects that helps you diminish pain. It's reasonable to hold at this dose for a while, let your body adjust, and then decide whether or not you want to go to an even lower dose. You may not feel comfortable totally discontinuing your opioid medications, at least not at this time, which is fine for now. You can stay at this dose, or at a later date when you feel ready, decrease the dose even more. I strongly believe it will be easier to wean off medications after you have done some of the exercises in this book.

Alternatively, with close medical supervision, you can stop your medications, substituting the medications listed with the addition of tramadol or Suboxone for a brief period of time. I must stress that this needs to be accomplished by an experienced medical provider and would be done optimally in an inpatient setting. If you are using other substances (such as alcohol, sedatives, or stimulants), the detoxification will be more complicated and potentially dangerous and will require consultation with an experienced addiction specialist or physician who is knowledgeable and skilled in dealing with complex withdrawal.

Length of time in treatment for detoxification varies and is based on the symptoms that occur as the drug is discontinued. The symptoms will vary according to the dose and type of drug you are taking. For example, high-dose, long-acting methadone or fentanyl detoxification can take as long as fourteen days or more, whereas detox from moderate doses of hydrocodone or oxycodone typically takes less time, perhaps as few as five to seven days. A quality treatment center will individualize the detox process and work to diminish symptoms and stabilize patients so they have the best chance of sustaining the abstinent state. And remember—detox is only the first step along the path of pain recovery.

REASONABLE GOALS

Whatever you decide to do and wherever you choose to begin, by all means set reasonable objectives and expectations for yourself. As a general suggestion, you might consider beginning with just one or two modest goals for the first week. Then, over a period of a few weeks, return to the menu and consider adding and/or trying a new technique. By the end of the first month, you will have a wide range of healing methods and exercises that help reduce your pain and increase your self-confidence in managing your daily life. Or you may decide to concentrate your energies on one particular "point of balance" (mental, physical, emotional, or spiritual) that resonates with your particular needs at the moment or where you believe you need the most help. The important point is to get started, which is the purpose of the Jump Start Plan.

One of the most common issues that comes up at LVRC is the desire to improve rapidly, which can lead to impatience with slow gains. Mike, a former Olympic skier, expressed his frustration one day in group. "I'm so much better, I just want to be able to exercise like I used to when I was in training." Mike and I had a good talk that day about pacing and the art of moving forward at a slow, steady pace—walking for a few days, then fast walking, then jogging and, after a few weeks, running sprints on the treadmill.

After the first day of jogging, Mike found himself gasping for air. He was deeply discouraged. "I don't understand why I'm so out of shape," he said. "I used to be able to run ten miles without getting even a little winded."

"That was then, this is now, and you've been through a lot since then," I reminded him. "You're likely to get more strength and stamina back over time if you go slow and pace yourself."

Mike disciplined himself to slow down, build his endurance gradually, and ramp up to increased activity that brought him back to what he called "decent shape." Now, eight months later, he's training for a marathon.

THE ABSOLUTE ESSENTIALS

The Jump Start Plan offered in this chapter includes an extensive menu of healing methods for you to choose from. If you incorporate just one strategy a week, that is fine; if you want to try more, that is fine, too, as long as you don't overdo it. You are in charge. You are not asking a doctor or a family member to manage your care—you are taking control and making the decisions yourself. That approach, in and of itself, is healing. Patients who take responsibility for their well-being tend to do better. Of course, you cannot control everything, but you are in charge of your attitude and your willingness to change what you can. The work you put in *will* have an impact on your life.

I need to emphasize that of all the techniques and tools offered in this chapter, three are absolutely essential: nutrition, exercise, and sleep. Be sure to revisit the detailed sections on exercise and sleep in Chapter 6. Good nutrition is so important that I devote the next chapter to an in-depth discussion of healthy, pain-reducing foods (as well as discussing foods that can aggravate pain). Try to build in a walk every day, even if it is just a slow stroll from one room to the next (for some people that is the most exercise they've had in a very long time). As I mentioned before, if you exercise before four p.m. rather than closer to bedtime, you are likely to sleep better.

Sleep is one of the biggest challenges for patients in treatment, especially when coming off high doses of mood-altering drugs. In her book *The Recovering Body*, Jennifer Matesa explains:

> If there was one problem I faced during detox that made me want to go back to using drugs . . . it was lack of sleep . . . When our sleep tanks, the rest of life can tank: work performance, relationships, other health conditions. For addicts with chronic pain, this can be a recipe for a relapse. Which is why, when some recovering addicts I knew assured me blithely that "no one ever died from lack of sleep," I decided that anyone who could say this to a newly sober addict had to be a total asshat completely ignorant.

Sleep is absolutely essential because you cannot focus, concentrate, or make healthy decisions if you're not getting enough rest. But with a nutritious diet, a little bit of exercise, and a good night's sleep, many things are possible. Because you are human, pain is inevitable—but when you are able to manage your pain with a daily routine including healthy food, regular exercise, and sufficient rest, practiced with dedication and diligence, your self-confidence will increase and—I promise you—your pain will lessen.

The Jump Start Plan begins with these three essentials and also includes acupressure points that you can massage yourself (with specific advice on locations and techniques—see pages 155–157); breathing exercises that increase the oxygen available to your cells, which improves physical energy, invigorates thought processes, calms emotions, and settles the spirit (as explained on pages 171–174); reflections that can be used to start or end your day; and additional complementary and alternative medicine (CAMs) treatment approaches that easily can be added into your weekly routine.

Incorporate as many of the following changes as you can into your daily routine. And, as always, be gentle with yourself. Don't rush into anything and don't pressure yourself with self-defeating thoughts, such as "This is too much, it's too overwhelming!" or "I'm not working on this as hard as I should be." (If thoughts like these run through your mind, go back to Chapter 5, page 119, and do a thought pattern chart, assessing whether your thoughts are irrational or reasonable.)

Proceed at your own pace, picking and choosing what you think might be most helpful. If it takes you a year to include several strategies outlined in the Jump Start Plan, then that's what it takes! And like so many people, you might discover that just two or three techniques work wonders for you. Keep the remaining recommendations in hand, though, in case you need additional support.

Most important of all is to keep in mind that you are in charge—no one else. Being thorough and methodical is just as effective as being gung-ho and trying everything. Remind yourself and others that this is a process and that you are in control. I give you permission right now to refrain from judging yourself. And I suggest that you tell others who might be subtly or overtly critical of your progress to just "let you be" as you move along this pathway.

That said, I recommend meeting with a health coach, in conjunction with your doctor, to review your individualized Jump Start Plan and offer additional ideas or suggestions. Alternative medicine practitioners, including naturopathic physicians, physical therapists, acupuncturists, massage therapists, and yoga teachers, can offer valuable advice as well.

As the ancient Chinese sage Lao-tzu wrote, "The journey of a thousand miles begins with a single step." Every step counts.

Four-Week Jump Start Plan

	Week 1	Week 2 Add to Week 1	Week 3 Add to Weeks 1 & 2	Week 4 Add to Weeks 1, 2 & 3
Diet/ nutrition	1. Drink 8 glasses of water daily. 2. Omega-3 supplement 3. Vitamin D supplement	Begin to cut back on "anti-nutrients"— caffeine, refined sugar, fructose, and sugar-rich foods.	Increase consumption of fruits and vegetables (gently steam vegetables).	Reduce red meat consumption to 1–2 times/ week; add more fish to your diet.
Exercise	Gentle stretching (5 minutes, twice daily)	Walk 5–10 minutes daily (if not possible, return to Week One's routine and build up over the next 2 weeks).	Increase walks to 15–20 minutes. Gentle aerobic exercise (again, if possible to increase to this level).	Swimming, bicycling, treadmill, or elliptical (15–30 minutes per day if you are able)
Sleep	If you nap, limit to 5- to 10-minute "power naps" (or try Shavasana, page 182).	Set a consistent time for going to sleep and getting up in the morning.	Avoid large, late meals; if hungry before bed, eat a "sleep-aid" snack (banana, hot chamomile tea, warm milk).	Keep a sleep diary by your bed, noting troublesome thoughts or dreams.
Acupoint	Large Intestine 4: "Great Eliminator" (page 155)	Liver 3: "Great Rushing" (page 156)	Kidney 3: "Great Mountain Stream" (page 157)	Conception Vessel 4: "Sea of Energy" (page 157)
Breathing exercises	Calming Breath (page 172)	Belly Breath (page 172)	Prana Breath (page 173)	Breathing *Om* (page 173)
Reflection (journaling)	"What am I afraid of losing?"	"Why do I deserve to be loved and supported?"	"What benefits do I get from my pain?"	"What can I control in my life? What can't I control?"
If you are so moved, try . . .	Massage	Yoga class	Chi Kung or Tai Chi class	Acupuncture session

Modifying Your Jump Start Plan

If you are reading this book, the chances are good that you are either living with chronic pain or you love someone in chronic pain. Chronic pain is our common denominator. And yet even as we share similar thoughts, feelings, and experiences, we are all unique. Certain steps or strategies will resonate with your energy level and emotional or spiritual needs, while other techniques may not appeal to you—at least in the early stages of establishing a self-management routine.

Your unique Jump Start Plan will also vary according to your particular diagnosis (chronic low back pain, arthritis, head or neck pain, fibromyalgia, chronic fatigue syndrome, peripheral neuropathy, for example) and any complicating diseases or disorders you might need to address, such as allergies, asthma, sinusitis, diabetes, cancer, heart disease, lung disease, HIV/AIDS and other chronic infections, and many more.

MONTH 2 JUMP START PLANS

Here are Jump Start Plans for five common chronic pain conditions. If you have low back pain, arthritis, fibromyalgia or chronic fatigue syndrome, migraines, or neuropathy, you will find additional healing tips and techniques in this section. Follow the Jump Start Plan on page 217 for the first four weeks and then begin to incorporate some of the suggestions for your particular type of chronic pain.

Low Back Pain

JUMP START PLAN—MONTH 2

Low back pain is the most common type of chronic pain. Symptoms include shooting or stabbing pain; pain that radiates down your leg; limited flexibility or range of motion of the back; and, in severe cases, the inability to stand up straight. Chronic low back pain may be caused by muscle or ligament strain; bulging or ruptured disks; osteoarthritis in the spine, which can lead to spinal stenosis (narrowing of the space around the spinal cord); skeletal irregularities, such as scoliosis (curving of the spine); and osteoporosis (when your bones become porous and brittle), leading to compression fractures of the spine's vertebrae.

One of the most common diagnoses for chronic low back pain is degenerative disk disease, which is the equivalent of wrinkles on the skin—wear and tear from living life in an upright position.

Phil, 33, has been home for ten days after spending a month in treatment for low back pain related to a rugby injury, as well as detox and treatment for addiction to Percocet and morphine. His back pain periodically flares up, although he now rates the pain as a 2 or 3 on the 10-point scale, rather than the 8 or 9 he reported before treatment. While his craving for opioids has abated, he sometimes experiences an intense desire to use again, usually in midmorning or late afternoon. He is careful to eat three healthy meals and he's discovered that having a snack two or three times a day (almonds, fruit, gluten-free crackers, and cheese) helps keep his cravings under control.

Phil follows his counselor's advice to attend Narcotics Anonymous meetings, but he hasn't been able to find a group where he feels as if he fits and belongs. He decides to try AA meetings instead and, for some reason, they seem to suit him better. He makes a list of all the AA meetings in town and sets out to keep his commitment (part of his written discharge plan) to attend four or five meetings every week. After attending three different meetings, he finds one he really likes. "I can't explain it, I just felt at home the minute I walked into the room," he told me. From that point on, he has faithfully attended five meetings every week and sometimes adds a Saturday or Sunday meeting.

The 1-2-3 Plan for Low Back Pain

When my low back pain flares up, I am not a happy guy. I don't sleep well, I find work difficult, movement aggravates the pain, I get cranky, irritable, and I don't like myself very much as a result. Here's a 1-2-3 strategy I use to prevent my back from getting the best of me. You can do all three steps if you have the time and inclination or choose just one (and save the others for later in the day if your back is still acting up).

continues

continued

1. **Breathe:** I step away from what I am doing, sit or lie down with my eyes closed, and take a deep breath. Holding my breath, I count to seven, and then exhale to a count of eight. I bring my awareness to my low back, noticing how tight and knotted the muscles are, and for the next three inhalations and exhalations, I send cleansing breaths to those areas.
2. **Stretch:** I bend forward, letting my back stretch, and then rise up and clasp my hands behind my back, expanding my chest, arching my back, and breathing. I repeat this three times.
3. **Get out of myself:** My pain is always greater when I am thinking about it, so I "get out of myself" by calling or talking to someone. At work I often talk to a patient or write an e-mail to former patients. In the evenings or on weekends, I call a good friend. Sometimes I say a quick prayer ("Please take this pain away in this moment"), turning to a force greater than myself for help.

Four-Week Jump Start Plan—Month 2 for Back Pain

	Week 5	Week 6 Add to Week 5	Week 7 Add to Weeks 5 & 6	Week 8 Add to Weeks 5, 6 & 7
Diet/ nutrition	Water can reduce muscle spasms and inflammation—drink lots of it!	Spice up your meals with garlic, turmeric, and ginger—all are powerful and safe anti-inflammatories.	Magnesium—found in beans, seeds, nuts, avocados, bananas and dark green, leafy vegetables—helps relax and contract muscles and maintain muscle tone and bone density.	Tart cherries, strawberries, raspberries, blueberries, and blackberries will help your body control inflammation.

continues

Four-Week Jump Start Plan—Month 2 for Back Pain *continued*

	Week 5	Week 6 Add to Week 5	Week 7 Add to Weeks 5 & 6	Week 8 Add to Weeks 5, 6 & 7
Exercise	Make a commitment to exercise *every day*. Stretching is especially beneficial for back pain.	Hamstring stretches—standing up, bend from the waist and try to touch your toes—don't strain!	Yoga poses will help with flexibility and strength—consider taking a gentle yoga class (also see Resources for recommended books).	Combine acupressure (try Large Intestine 4, page 155) with a focused breathing technique (Calming Breath or Prana Breath, pages 172–173).
Sleep	Try relaxation techniques—the body scan meditation can be very helpful for low back pain.	Keep a worry diary or journal on your bedside table.	If you have trouble falling asleep or if you wake up in the night, try free-writing.	Buy a sleep-inducing CD (see Resources for suggestions).
Reflection (journaling or meditating)	"Pain is fleeting—what can I focus on that is constant and unchanging?"	"What do I fear? Where do I tend to store my fear?"	"What is the object of my anger? How can I effectively express my anger?"	"What do I need to let go of—why am I holding on?"
If you are so moved, try . . .	Heat and ice: Ice packs to reduce inflammation and heat therapy to stimulate blood flow. Both heat and ice inhibit relay of pain messages.	The 1-2-3 Plan (see pages 219–220).	Tennis Ball Massage: Use two tennis balls, each wrapped in a sock. Lie down and place a sock on either side of your spine, shifting your weight to massage your back.	Attend several recovery support groups (AA, NA, PIRSG, grief groups) and find one where you feel you "fit and belong."

A Warning About Spinal Surgery

If you have chronic back pain, you may be thinking about surgery.

Before considering spinal surgery investigate all other options and always, always, always get a second opinion.

My esteemed colleague Dr. David Hanscom is a spinal surgeon who recently wrote an editorial titled "Spine Surgery Is Just One Tool—Not the 'Definitive Answer.'" The long-term "success rate" for low back surgery is less than 30 percent and the risks (additional surgery, increased pain, lifetime disability) are very high. As Dr. Hanscom writes:

> Research shows that over half the patients have significant improvement at six months out from a LBP [lower back pain] fusion, but at two year follow up this number has dropped to less than 30%. Additionally, the re-operation rate is 15–20% within the first year, there is over a 30% chance of having increased pain after surgery, and even a higher chance that you may enter the terrible reality of becoming a "failed back surgery syndrome" patient. Being part of this group means that you will be condemned to suffer crippling pain the rest your life. Your capacity to thrive and enjoy your life shrinks to less than zero and your life becomes one of just surviving the adversity caused by pain.

Arthritis

JUMP START PLAN—MONTH 2

Arthritis is a general term that covers more than a hundred different joint diseases. About 52.5 million Americans have arthritis. Osteoarthritis is the most common type of arthritis and occurs when the cartilage covering the bones starts to wear away or degenerate with age or overuse so that the bones rub against each other, leading to pain and swelling.

Julio, 41, has rheumatoid arthritis. The onset of the disease was subtle and gradual. Julio began to notice that his knees and ankles were stiff in the morning, but he didn't pay a lot of attention as the pain tended to dissipate when he started moving around. "I'm just getting a little older," he told his concerned wife, "and being on my feet all day in my teaching job isn't helping things." Over the next few years the stiffness became more widespread, with throbbing and at times stabbing pains in his knees, hands, wrists, and fingers, affecting his ability to write and walk.

Julio refused to take prescription painkillers because he feared becoming dependent upon them. For years he managed the pain with ibuprofen, but when the swelling and stiffness increased and interfered with his work, he decided to see his doctor. Honoring Julio's desire to stay away from opioid drugs, his doctor suggested that he try the Jump Start Plans outlined in this chapter. In the first month Julio lost 5 pounds, his energy improved, and his pain lessened. Following the Month 2 Jump Start Plan for Arthritis, he found that cutting out red meat and other animal fats—and eliminating his traditional 16-ounce glass of orange juice in the morning—significantly reduced his symptoms. To the surprise of his wife and co-workers, he enrolled in a gentle yoga class and began his own yoga practice at home, incorporating yoga stretches and breathing exercises into his daily morning and evening routine.

Recently Julio purchased a hot tub. At night, after work, he enjoys sitting in the hot tub and on weekends he "doubles up," with an extra hot-tub soak in the morning. "Sure, I have pain, but I have all these new things in my life that help me deal with it and give me a lot of joy," he says. "I'm in better shape, so far I've lost fifteen pounds, yoga is a lot of fun, and I love soaking in the hot tub with my wife. Life is better than good."

Ginger Foot Bath

Ginger is an ancient "warming" remedy traditionally used to relieve nausea and vomiting. A ginger foot bath will help with circulatory problems, aches and pains in the legs or lower back, insomnia, and tense or bunched-up muscles. As an alternative, try a full bath to help you perspire and release toxins—just toss 2 to 6 tablespoons of powdered ginger in the tub as it's filling up.

1. Fill a small basin or rubber tub with comfortably hot water. Make sure the tub is large enough to fit both your feet!
2. Add enough water to cover your feet up to your ankles.

continues

continued

3. Stir 1 to 2 tablespoons of ground ginger or ¼ cup of grated fresh ginger into the water, mixing with your hands to dissolve.
4. Play some soothing music, read a book, and sip a glass of water while you relax and enjoy the foot bath. You might also want to light a candle or two!
5. Soak for 15 minutes or more. (Don't worry about wrinkly feet!) If the water cools off, add more warm water.
6. Pat your feet dry with a soft towel and take a few calming breaths.

Jump Start Plan—Month 2 for Arthritis

	Week 5	Week 6 Add to Week 5	Week 7 Add to Weeks 5 & 6	Week 8 Add to Weeks 5, 6 & 7
Diet/ nutrition	Avoid red meat, poultry, and animal fats, which can inflame your joints.	Cut back or eliminate "nightshade" veggies (eggplant, peppers, tomatoes, potatoes).	Avoid oranges and orange juice (the acids in oranges can irritate delicate joint membranes).	Take 1,500 mg of gamma linoleic acid (GLA), which has anti-inflammatory properties.
Exercise	Swim or exercise in a heated pool.	Take a gentle yoga class.	Walk as often as possible outside in the fresh air.	Walk on a treadmill when the weather keeps you indoors.
Sleep	Give yourself a gentle, soothing "head massage" (page 229).	Consider purchasing a memory foam pillow.	Reduce the weight of your blankets or comforters (lightweight down comforters are a great choice).	Take a hot (but not too hot) bath an hour or two before bedtime.
Reflection (journaling or meditating)	"How do I resist change in my life?"	"Where am I blocked creatively?"	"Am I turning my anger, fear, and anxiety against myself?"	"How can I learn to stand up for myself and assert myself with clarity and force?"
If you are so moved, try . . .	Ginger Foot Bath (see box, pages 223–224).	Physical therapy (passive exercises to increase mobility and flexibility).	Massage (Rolfing can be particularly helpful).	Ginger tea (see recipe, page 272).

Fibromyalgia and Chronic Fatigue Syndrome

JUMP START PLAN—MONTH 2

Most experts believe that chronic fatigue syndrome and fibromyalgia have a common underlying cause and may represent the same underlying disorder. The symptoms are similar in both disorders—chronic, debilitating fatigue and loss of energy, often described as "drop-dead flu"—and treatments that prove effective for one condition turn out to be effective for the other. Fibromyalgia is an example of "central sensitization" discussed in Chapter 2, when the volume in the brain's pain center is turned up. After following the Jump Start Plan on page 217 for four weeks, begin to incorporate some of the suggestions in this section.

Lynn was diagnosed with fibromyalgia at age twenty-two. She was actually relieved when the arthritis specialist gave her the diagnosis, because she finally had an explanation for the chronic fatigue and sensitivity to touch that had plagued her for the last ten years. Unfortunately she had already started on a hefty dose of oxymorphone (a strong opioid) for the awful, aching pain that aggravated her every waking moment. The drug dulled the pain for a while, but it always came back with a vengeance. The medication also made her edgy and depressed, and she spent more and more time in a dark room, watching TV. The more she moved, the more her body hurt—so she simply stopped moving. Her doctor also prescribed Valium for anxiety and to help her sleep. "The only time I get total relief from the pain," she told me, "is when I am asleep."

Lynn eventually became so fed up with feeling sick and tired and watching her life slip away that she consulted a homeopathic doctor and began working with a nutritionist and exercise therapist. They all agreed that because she wasn't moving, her condition kept getting worse, and she embarked on a series of changes in her life associated with the following Jump Start Plan. She noticed improvements almost immediately when she was able to decrease the medications under her addiction doctor's watchful eye and "get moving again." By Week 7 she was completely off meds, taking two walks a day, and proudly announced that she felt like her old self again.

Jump Start Plan—Month 2 for Fibromyalgia

	Week 5	Week 6 Add to Week 5	Week 7 Add to Weeks 5 & 6	Week 8 Add to Weeks 5, 6 & 7
Diet/ nutrition	Schedule an appointment with a physician or nutritionist to assess possible food allergies.	Avoid red meat and dairy products and eat only *organic* fish and chicken; choose "wild" fish over farm-raised fish, if possible.	Limit or eliminate sugar, honey, corn syrup, and sugar substitutes.	Avoid fried, greasy, and highly processed foods; and avoid caffeine, which paradoxically drains energy from your depleted system.
Exercise	Avoid strenuous exercise.	Walk 5 minutes twice a day.	Increase walks to 10 minutes twice a day.	Sign up for a gentle yoga, Chi Kung, or Tai Chi class.
Sleep	Check with your doctor to make sure anemia and/or thyroid problems are not contributing to your fatigue.	Snoring, sleep apnea, allergies, or respiratory problems may be interfering with your sleep. Again, your health-care practitioner can help assess these problems.	Make your bedroom sleep-friendly—limit noise, light, and other stimuli (such as pets).	Consider purchasing hyper-allergenic bedding if you suffer from allergies of any kind.
Reflection (journaling or meditation)	"What makes me feel sick and tired?"	"How can I bring more joy and enthusiasm into my life?"	"How do my symptoms help me pay attention to myself and my needs?"	"What do my symptoms prevent me from doing, accomplishing, or being?"
If you are so moved, try . . .	Check out the National Fibromyalgia Association website (fmaaware.org)	Sinus Cleanse (see page 227)	Try massage and/or acupuncture treatments with a qualified professional	Astragalus, a Chinese herb used to support the immune system and promote energy (seek advice from a qualified herbalist)

Sinus Cleanse

Allergies and chronic sinus infections can complicate or exacerbate all types of chronic pain. Periodic sinus cleanses may help calm down a hyperreactive immune system and ease your symptoms. Many drugstores carry inexpensive sinus rinse kits, but it's easy (and much cheaper) to use this "recipe."

1. Put a teaspoon of sea salt and a pinch of baking soda in a cup of luke-warm water. Use distilled or purified (boiled, then cooled) water.
2. Mix well and pour a small amount of the solution into the cupped palm of your hand (or you can use a Neti pot).
3. Gently inhale through one nostril, moving your head around to circulate the saltwater solution.
4. Let the water drain out of your nose or spit it out of your mouth.
5. Gargle with the remaining solution, and spit it out.
6. Follow this routine once a day.

Migraine Headaches

JUMP START PLAN—MONTH 2

Migraine ranks in the top 20 of the world's most disabling medical illnesses, according to the Migraine Research Foundation. Eighteen percent of American women and 6 percent of men—about 36 million people in the United States—suffer from recurring migraine.

Susan has chronic migraine headaches. She loves to read and write and decides to drive to a local bookstore rather than order a book on-line. She parks her car a block from the store and walks slowly, taking care to breathe with each step. Deep breathing, she knows from following the first month Jump Start Plan, can alleviate her chronic headaches and even prevent them from occurring. Before she entered inpatient treatment, she was having three or four headaches per week but now, eight weeks later, she hasn't had a migraine for over a month. The thought of writing a full page in a journal overwhelms her, so she chooses a five-year journal that limits her to just five lines daily. "I can handle that," she thinks. For the next two weeks, she writes in her

Jump Start Plan—Month 2 for Migraine

	Week 5	Week 6 Add to Week 5	Week 7 Add to Weeks 5 & 6	Week 8 Add to Weeks 5, 6 & 7
Diet/ nutrition	Be sure to drink lots of water, especially if you feel a headache coming on.	Flax- and chia seeds are high in omega-3s and can fight the inflammation that causes headaches.	Ginger has anti-inflammatory properties and can ease migraine-related nausea.	Small doses of caffeine can sometimes help with headaches, but too much caffeine can trigger them.
Exercise	Avoid strenuous exercise, which dilates blood vessels and can trigger headaches.	Focus on gentle daily exercises—walking, stretching, yoga, swimming.	Breathing exercises can help relieve stress and tension; try the "Calming Breath."	Sign up for a gentle yoga, Chi Kung, or Tai Chi class.
Sleep	Establish consistent bed and wake times.	Create a dark, quiet, distraction-free sleep space (no TV, cell phone, alarm clock).	Avoid alcohol, nicotine, and caffeine, all of which interfere with a good night's sleep.	Before you go to bed, practice relaxation techniques and calming activities (heart-racing TV shows or books are not recommended).
Reflection (journaling or meditation)	"What obstacles confront me and what can I do to break through them?"	"I feel confined, trapped, imprisoned: What can I do to break free?"	"I have difficulty expressing myself: What fears prevent me from expressing myself openly?"	"I am often critical of others: What can I do to become more tolerant of other people's flaws and imperfections?"
If you are so moved, try . . .	Feverfew tea or supplements (or even chewing on this herb's leaves) can help ward off migraines.	Biofeedback is proven to help with headaches—give it a try.	Head Massage (see page 229)	Take a hot bath, then put an ice pack wrapped in a towel on your forehead (paradoxical relief).

journal every night before bed. In Week 3, she takes another look at the Month 2 Jump Start Plan for Migraines and decides to substitute ginger tea for her morning coffee, along with a hot bath followed by a cold pack, wrapped in a towel, on her forehead. She also makes an appointment with a masseuse who, friends tell her, "has a healing touch."

Head Massage

1. Place your thumbs just behind your ears.
2. Put the four other fingers of both hands on either side of the middle of your scalp with the pinkies at your hairline.
3. Using firm, steady pressure, press your fingertips into your scalp.
4. Slowly move your hands backward to the base of the skull, stopping every inch or so to apply firm pressure.
5. Return to the hairline, placing your fingers about an inch below your hairline and repeat the massage, moving down to the base of the skull and back up again.
6. Keep moving your fingers down your head until you've massaged your whole scalp.
7. If you feel any sensitive spots, spend extra time massaging those areas.

This entire exercise should take just three to four minutes.

Peripheral Neuropathy

JUMP START PLAN—MONTH 2

Peripheral neuropathy results from damage to the nerve itself and can cause numbness, weakness, and pain, as well as tingling, burning, or squeezing ("like a tight stocking compressing my feet") sensations. Peripheral neuropathy can affect people with diabetes, physical injuries (trauma), alcoholism, multiple sclerosis, kidney disorders, connective tissue disorders, infections (including HIV/AIDS, Lyme disease, and hepatitis), autoimmune disorders, cancers and benign tumors. Environmental toxins and certain medications, including anti-cancer drugs, anti-convulsants, anti-viral agents, and antibiotics, can also cause peripheral nerve damage. Up to 30 percent of chronic neuropathic pain is of unknown origin.

Like 60 to 70 percent of all people diagnosed with type 2 diabetes, Anthony has peripheral neuropathy. Chronically high blood sugar levels damaged the nerves in his hands and feet, causing pain and numbness. Anthony has worked hard to follow his doctor's treatment regimen, but he is finding it difficult to give up his "only remaining pleasures"—diet soda and potato chips. After following the initial Four-Week Jump Start Plan and acknowledging to his wife and doctor that he had more energy and less pain, Anthony makes a commitment to make additional changes in his life.

In Week 1 of the Month 2 Jump Start Plan for neuropathy, he decided simply to notice when he drank soda and ate chips and to write down what he was thinking and feeling at these times. In Week 6, he agreed to investigate alternatives and discovered that unsalted, gluten-free pretzels and a splash of cranberry juice mixed with carbonated water satisfied his "chips and soda" cravings. In Week 7 he completely eliminated soda from his diet and discovered a natural brand of "veggie chips" that he liked. "Who would have imagined that vegetables could taste so good?" he said, reporting that he had also lost several pounds and was thinking about substituting "real" vegetables (carrots and celery) for the chips. In Week 8 he decided to listen to a relaxation CD for five or ten minutes a day.

Jump Start Plan—Month 2 for Neuropathy

	Week 5	Week 6 Add to Week 5	Week 7 Add to Weeks 5 & 6	Week 8 Add to Weeks 5, 6 & 7
Diet/ nutrition	Eliminate sugary foods (candy, sweets, soft drinks) from your diet.	Try a gluten-free diet, replacing wheat and "white" bread and pasta products with oats, brown rice, and quinoa.	Cut back or eliminate dairy products.	Gradually eliminate red meat from your diet and add fatty fish (salmon, sardines, herring, mackerel, bluefish, albacore tuna).

continues

	Week 5	Week 6 Add to Week 5	Week 7 Add to Weeks 5 & 6	Week 8 Add to Weeks 5, 6 & 7
Exercise	Exercise daily but gently to improve blood flow (20–30 minutes daily).	Non-weight-bearing activities: swimming or bicycling (stationary bikes or arm cycles are great for strength and tone)	Light aerobics using free weights in a seated position	Chi Kung (can be done sitting or even lying down) or gentle yoga
Sleep	Quit smoking! If you cannot quit right away, do not smoke before bedtime or in the middle of the night. Continue your efforts to quit smoking until you succeed.	Limit or eliminate caffeine—no caffeine at all four to six hours before bed.	Give yourself an extra hour before bed to relax and unwind.	Keep a "worry journal" by your bed and write down any troubling thoughts or concerns.
Reflection (journaling or meditation)	"When the pain comes and goes with no rhyme or reason, where can I turn for balance in my life?"	"What is the worst thing that could happen to me if I let my feelings out?"	"How do I allow fear to rule my life? What exactly do I fear and why?"	"What can I do to break through the obstacles confronting me?"
If you are so moved, try . . .	Foot Massage (see page 232)	Capsaicin creams (ArthriCare, Zostrix, others) may help relieve neuropathic pain. Read directions carefully.	Gingko and alpha lipoic acid (ALA) may help to reduce symptoms of neuropathy. Ask your doctor for advice when using any herbal or dietary supplement.	Using a TENS unit and/or biofeedback techniques may help relieve chronic neuropathic pain.

Toward the end of Month 2, Anthony reluctantly agreed to give meditation a try, choosing to sit on a comfy couch on his sunny back porch with his feet on an ottoman. Five minutes was plenty for him, at first, but after several days, he was able to "sit" for seven minutes and practice "just breathing." He plans to quit smoking for good ("Okay, okay," he told his doctor with a laugh, "I guess I had three 'remaining pleasures'"), and as a first step he consulted with his local American Lung Association program (see Resources, page 296) to find out about smoking cessation classes.

Foot Massage

1. Rub moisturizing lotion, massage oil, or plain old vegetable oil on your fingers. For a special treat, use peppermint- or lavender-scented oils.
2. Using both hands, squeeze your right foot, moving the pressure from your ankle to your toe.
3. Squeeze any sore spots for 10 to 20 seconds.
4. Press the sole, just beneath the ball of your foot, for 20 seconds.
5. Gently pull the toes apart, and with your fingers roll each toe back and forth several times.
6. Repeat the massage with your left foot.

This entire exercise should take just three to four minutes.

The Jump Start Plans in this chapter offer a "menu" of healing strategies and techniques. Initially, you will most likely try the methods that are most familiar to you and comfortable for you. As the days and weeks go by, stretch yourself a bit. Reiki may sound "weird," but do some research and see what other chronic pain patients are saying about its effectiveness or try a session and see how it feels. Acupressure is simple and easy—but ask around for a good acupuncturist and give a professional acupuncture session a try. Breathing techniques may prove helpful at first, but meditation? Nudge yourself—give it a try even if it's slightly out of your comfort zone!

Once you've dipped your toes into the healing waters of these tried-and-true techniques and witnessed the benefits, no matter how small, you will be motivated to do a little more . . . and then a little more . . . until you find that a whole new world has opened up before you. You will eventually experience this as your new "normal." And you have so much more to discover from here!

The Vital Role of Diet and Nutrition

In this chapter I've only touched on the profound importance of nutrition in the daily management of chronic pain. "You are what you eat" is an oft-repeated truism, but because certain foods aggravate chronic pain while other foods alleviate pain, Kathy and I decided that we needed an entire chapter to highlight the long-term health benefits of good nutrition. In the next chapter you will find a detailed nutritional program with dozens of tips and strategies to help you with what I consider to be one of the most important aspects of chronic pain recovery—choosing foods, beverages, menus, and meal plans that promote health and healing, while avoiding foods and other substances that can exacerbate your pain. In the Appendix (pages 265–292) you will find dozens of delicious (and, most important, easy) recipes to get you started.

Pay close attention to small improvements in your pain levels and sense of well-being. The goal is to work around the edges of the pain. Chipping off 5 to 10 percent with each of these modalities will decrease your pain significantly.

TEN

EATING RIGHT TO REDUCE YOUR PAIN

Foods That Hurt and Foods That Heal

Feeding yourself well, naturally, wholesomely,
and in balance will provide all the nutrients that
you need to nourish your whole self.

—ELSON HAAS, MD

Tart cherries, cranberries, spinach, red peppers, white tea, green tea, extra-virgin olive oil, salmon, grass-fed beef, free-range chicken, nuts, seeds, and—yes!—chocolate are all good choices for reducing inflammation and relieving pain. In this chapter you will learn about these and many more natural, wholesome foods. You will discover how short-term changes can lead to long-term gains. And you will find that healthy eating has a direct impact not just on your body, but on your mind, your emotions, and your ability to experience joy in everyday life. Being conscious and aware of your food choices, learning which foods make you feel better, trying different and unusual foods, and gaining confidence in your ability to follow a truly healthy diet are just a few of the benefits you will gain as you read and absorb the information in this chapter.

Ben's story offers an example of the interplay between the food we eat, the weight we gain (or lose), and the pain we feel. His journey began when he was diagnosed with ulcers. Medications quickly consumed his life and almost ended it.

BEN'S STORY

At age thirty-two, Ben started to have chronic gastrointestinal problems involving abdominal cramping and heartburn. His doctor told him he had duodenal ulcers, open sores or lesions in the upper portion of the small intestine.

For the next three years Ben's health went downhill. His stomach was constantly upset and even small amounts of food made him nauseous. He lost weight and looked pale and emaciated. One day he woke up in agony. He felt he could barely breathe because of the razor-sharp pain.

The emergency room doctor told him the ulcer had become so large that surgery was required. After the operation, Ben was given prescriptions for 40 mg of Vicodin and 30 mg of Valium per day. When Ben came home from the hospital, he was depressed, in pain, and anxious about his potential for a full recovery. Two months after the surgery, the pain was worse—8 out of 10 on the pain scale—and Ben was frustrated, scared, and even more depressed. His doctor was concerned and prescribed 150 mg of amitriptyline, an anti-depressant, and 4 mg of Ativan, another benzodiazepine drug for anxiety, in addition to the Valium. By then, Ben was up to 80 mg of Vicodin or more per day.

Five months after surgery, Ben rated his pain as 9 out of 10, and he admitted he was so depressed that he actively contemplated suicide. His doctor changed his anti-depressant, continued the anti-anxiety drugs, and added 40 mg of OxyContin three times per day for his increased level of pain.

Ben's wife and three daughters were frantic with worry. With his family's help and encouragement, he agreed to enter treatment.

When I initially examined him, Ben was in obvious emotional distress. He frequently broke down in tears, seemed on the edge of despair, and talked openly about killing himself. "My life has been pure misery ever since that damn surgery," he said. "I just need help. Please help me!" he pleaded.

Ben's blood work showed low calcium, low protein, anemia, and low thyroid function. Suspecting blood sugar abnormalities, I ordered a glucose tolerance test, which was highly abnormal with a quick sugar rise and a sudden plummet to 35 mg/dl (70–100 mg/dl is considered normal) during the second hour of the test, accompanied by symptoms of extreme fatigue and depression. His abnormally low blood sugar levels contributed to his anxiety and irritability. Ben was also low in vitamin D.

Ben's treatment started with detoxification from his medications. Because of the high doses and multiple drugs he was taking, detox lasted two weeks. In groups and individual sessions he learned about addiction and the dangers of taking potentially addictive prescription drugs. After consultation with the dietitian, nutritional therapy stabilized his blood sugar, corrected his calcium and vitamin D deficiencies, and began the job of repairing and restoring his health. Proper diet and supplements resulted in normal blood levels, and within a week he was physically feeling much better.

The first few weeks were a bit rocky, with his depression and emotional ups and downs only gradually decreasing. Ben's abdominal pain was a consistent problem, with cramps and diarrhea, but after a few more weeks, he was able to tolerate more and more foods without discomfort. He understood the need to avoid sugar and sugar-rich foods and created his own plan for avoiding hidden sugars in foods, such as coffee creamer, fruit yogurt, granola bars, and whole wheat bread.

After five weeks in treatment, Ben and his family couldn't believe the transformation in his physical, mental, emotional, and spiritual health. He practically glowed with good health and exuberant energy. After six weeks, he left treatment feeling healthy, happy, and firmly committed to his recovery and a drug-free life.

■ ■ ■

LET THY FOOD BE THY MEDICINE

Twenty-five hundred years ago, Hippocrates, the Father of Medicine, urged his students to "let thy food be thy medicine and thy medicine thy food." Hippocrates left no doubt about his objection to powerful drugs when he said, "Leave your drugs in the chemist's pot if you can heal the patient with food." Today's medical students receive a different message. As Neal Barnard, MD, writes in a 2014 article titled "Curing Doctors' Dangerous Lack of Nutrition Education":

Doctors learn about prescription drugs and about surgery. But the role of food is underemphasized in medical education. Currently, most patients who seek doctors' help for these problems only find a cocktail of drugs or a scalpel—approaches that continually fail to treat or heal. The vast majority of American doctors never learn that dietary approaches exist—so neither do their patients . . . Despite the prevalence of diet-related disease, the number of schools offering the minimum nutrition instruction is declining.

What did I learn about nutrition in medical school back in the 1970s? Here's a sad (and embarrassing) fact—I don't remember any lectures, courses, or reading assignments on diet and nutrition, except for learning about diabetes in my endocrinology class and a brief review of heart-healthy diets in my internal medicine rotation. As Dr. Barnard points out, even today medical students do not receive adequate education or information about the healing (and deleterious) effects of diet and nutrition. As a result, many physicians feel out of their element discussing nutrition, because this is an area outside their expertise.

The good news is that the entire health-care field is paying more attention to wellness and disease prevention these days, and many doctors and other health-care practitioners are educating themselves about nutrition and diet. Don't hesitate to ask your doctor for dietary advice and nutritional counseling. If he or she is unable to provide adequate information, ask for a referral. I also recommend meeting with a nutrition professional or health coach, in conjunction with your doctor, to learn how to balance your unique symptoms and develop a nutrition plan that is right for you. Alternative medicine practitioners, including physical therapists, acupuncturists, massage therapists, and yoga teachers, are often well-schooled in nutritional science and can offer valuable advice.

While Kathy and I are not experts in nutritional science, we work with people who are. With their help in this chapter, we seek to emphasize the critical importance of nutrition for long-term recovery from both chronic pain and chemical dependence. The remainder of this chapter represents our combined efforts to create general guidelines to healthy eating (and drinking) for people with chronic pain, along with lists of foods that can help reduce pain, foods to avoid, and tips to get you started (you'll find some wonderful recipes in the Appendix, pages 265–292). Rest assured that this "diet" is not designed for weight loss, although that can be one of its additional benefits. I do not ask you to count calories. Instead, these guidelines will help you focus on gaining, not losing—gaining valuable nutrients by eating the right kinds of food that can help reduce inflammation and alleviate pain.

The information in this chapter is merely an overview. The field of diet and nutrition is so vast and constantly evolving that I will touch only on the basics. Be sure to check out the Resources section, where you will find trustworthy books focusing specifically on nutritional advice for people living with chronic pain and/or in recovery from addiction to alcohol or other drugs.

About now, you may be groaning about having more work to do. Shopping, chopping, cooking, and even eating may rank low on your to-do list. "Lack of energy, lack of sleep, and constant pain—well, basically food gets shoved to the side," Sarah explains. "Often I'm in a rotten flare at dinner time and I couldn't whip up a bowl of cold cereal if my life depended on it. Flulike symptoms of fibromyalgia and loss of appetite caused by the pain are huge stumbling blocks for me. I just don't like food anymore. I don't like the taste, I don't like to cook, and I have to force myself to eat, so I often choose something quick and simple and usually not good for me."

The possibility of changing the eating habits of a lifetime might seem like an overwhelming task, and you may wonder whether subtle or even large-scale changes in your diet will have any significant impact on your pain. For the reluctant and the doubting, I suggest this plan: Follow the general principles of the food plan below for just one month. At the end of the month, judge how you feel, and if you find a significant reduction in your pain level and an improvement in your energy, emotional balance, state of mind, and physical well-being, make a longer-term commitment at that point. Let the results convince you that changing your dietary habits is worth the effort in terms of your general health and well-being.

GENERAL PRINCIPLES

Before we get to the specifics, here are some general, easy-to-follow principles:

PRINCIPLE 1: Keep it simple! Don't make the task of following these guidelines too difficult. Remember, you don't have to count calories or measure foods—and you never need to feel hungry!

Pain Reduction Diet—Weeks 1–4

	Week 1	Week 2	Week 3	Week 4
Keep it simple!	Eat 3 small meals, 3 small snacks a day.	Concentrate on "whole" foods.	Eat fish at least once a week.	Slowly eliminate starches (bread, rice, potatoes).
Water	Drink 8 glasses of water every day—and keep a water bottle by your desk or computer.	Use sliced lemons and cucumbers in water—the good taste will help you drink more!	When you feel hungry, try drinking a glass of water or two before eating.	Buy a water filter device and extra BPA-free bottles.
Breakfast	No more skipping breakfast!	Make a spinach omelet in your egg cooker.	Use your slow cooker to make Creamy Coconut Oatmeal (page 268).	Try a "green" smoothie with kale, spinach, and lots of fresh fruit—not bad!
Fresh fruits and veggies	Make a list of your favorite fruits and veggies.	Find a local source for organic fruits and veggies.	Learn how to freeze fruit and vegetables for winter meals.	Get adventurous—buy a mango and maybe a pomegranate!
Nutritious snacks	Make a list of nutritious snacks and star your favorites.	Try organic hummus with carrots and red pepper slices.	Apple slices dipped in almond butter (from health food store)	Natural peanut or almond butter on gluten-free crackers.
Sugar	Try almond milk in your coffee—naturally sweet!	Avoid morning and midday sweets (such as doughnuts and cookies).	Buy raw organic agave syrup to try in plain yogurt.	Give up desserts this week.
Refined and processed foods	Find healthy alternative to your vanilla-flavored coffee creamer!	Use the bread maker to make whole-grain bread.	Buy brown rice and always substitute for white rice.	Eat only gluten-free pasta.
Toxins	Inform your relatives who smoke cigarettes that your home is a smoke-free zone; ban e-cigs as well.	Clean cabinets of toxic chemicals—air fresheners, cleaning compounds, bug sprays.	Learn how to read labels for unhealthy additives and make a list of substances to avoid!	Plan a summer garden with lots of fruits and veggies—and no pesticides!

PRINCIPLE 2: **Drink plenty of water,** *at least* eight 8-ounce glasses every day (preferably filtered). Health coaches often recommend drinking 5 ounces per pound of body weight. Thus, if you weight 120, drink 75 ounces or about nine 8-ounce glasses daily; if you weigh 180, drink eleven 8-ounce glasses daily.

PRINCIPLE 3: **Eat breakfast!** There are many reasons not to skip this vitally important meal: Breakfast jump-starts your metabolism, helps you lose weight, increases your ability to concentrate and stay awake and alert, and improves your mood. Certified gluten-free oatmeal as well as millet, buckwheat, and quinoa are great choices for breakfast, as are eggs, nuts, and seeds. Add greens if you can—a spinach omelet or a green smoothie. Avoid packaged low-fat and nonfat foods, which contain extra sugar to take the place of the fat. Plain Greek yogurt sweetened with honey or raw organic agave syrup and sprinkled (or loaded) with pomegranate and chia seeds is one of Kathy's favorite breakfast meals, while oatmeal pancakes are my faithful standby (see recipe, page 270). Just so you know—I never leave the house without breakfast.

PRINCIPLE 4: **Add fresh fruits and veggies.** The newest recommendations from Harvard's Healthy Eating Plan call for eight portions of fruits and vegetables daily. If you have arthritis, avoid fruits and vegetables that can cause inflammation, including citrus fruits, potatoes, tomatoes, and corn. Certain fruits—apples and bananas, for example—can trigger headaches in susceptible people. You may have heard about the "Dirty Dozen Plus" fruits and veggies, which contain a high pesticide load and the "Clean 15," which contain the lowest pesticide load. Whenever possible, choose produce from the "Clean 15" or buy "100% organic" or "pesticide-free" (a label often used by local farmers) when choosing from the "Dirty Dozen Plus" list.

CLEAN 15
Foods that you don't have to buy "organic"

- Avocados
- Sweet corn
- Pineapples
- Cabbage
- Sweet peas (frozen)
- Onions

- Asparagus
- Mangoes
- Papayas
- Kiwi
- Eggplant

- Grapefruit
- Cantaloupe (domestic)
- Cauliflower
- Sweet potatoes

DIRTY DOZEN PLUS

- Apples
- Strawberries
- Grapes
- Celery
- Peaches
- Spinach

- Sweet bell peppers
- Nectarines (imported)
- Cucumbers
- Cherry tomatoes
- Snap peas (imported)
- Potatoes

Plus (produce that contains organosulfate insecticides, considered "highly toxic")

- Hot peppers

- Blueberries (domestic)

PRINCIPLE 5: **Add nutritious snacks** (three a day) to stabilize blood sugar and keep energy levels high. Choose from nutrient-rich fruits, seeds, and nuts (be aware that in susceptible people, nuts can trigger headaches, arthritis, and irritable bowel problems); high-protein foods, such as oatmeal, hummus, low-fat cottage cheese, or small portions of lean meat (chicken, turkey) or fish (tuna, salmon); and fruit (organic apples or grapes, cantaloupe slices) or veggie "sticks" (asparagus, organic celery or organic red, yellow, and green peppers).

PRINCIPLE 6: **Avoid sugar and sugar-laden foods.** We'll cover sugar in-depth in a moment, but for now: Read labels carefully and avoid foods that include the words *syrup*, *sweetener*, *sugar* (beet, brown, cane, coconut, palm, raw, rice), and anything ending in *ose*. Here are a few "code" words used on labels that you might not recognize as sugar: corn syrup, dextrose, dextrin, fructose, glucose, honey, lactose, malt syrup, maltose, maple syrup, molasses, sucrose, and xylose. Also avoid sugar substitutes, such as saccharine and aspartame. The jury is still out on stevia. I encourage you to learn to cook with honey, raw organic agave nectar, coconut sugar, or pure maple syrup, but in limited quantities.

PRINCIPLE 7: Cut way back on refined and processed foods. Refined foods, such as white flour, white rice, and white pasta products have little nutritious value, and processed meats (sausage, bacon, hot dogs, cold cuts) contain added salts and sugars in addition to sodium nitrates and other potentially harmful preservatives.

PRINCIPLE 8: Eliminate toxins. I consider toxins to be any substance (natural or man-made) that can damage your body (and therefore your mind and spirit), exacerbate your pain, and cause or accelerate disease. Chemicals and pesticides in food definitely qualify, so be sure to read labels. Tobacco is not a food, but let me state again that of all the offending toxins in this world, nicotine and tobacco smoke are the worst. *I strongly recommend that if you smoke or chew—QUIT!*

Toxins in Our Food

As you will see from the list below, you can't eliminate all toxins from your diet, but reading labels and choosing "whole" and "organic" foods will help.

- Pesticides (less likely to be found in organic foods, which are required to be free of synthetic pesticides)
- BHA (butylated hydroxyanisole) and BHT (butylated hydroxytoluene), food additives and preservatives found in cereals, snack foods, drink mixes, baked goods, chewing gum, instant mashed potatoes, and other foods
- Recombinant bovine growth hormone (rBGH/rBST), which you can avoid by using organic or rBGH-*free* dairy products
- Trans fats (formed in process of hydrogenation, found in margarine, shortening, spreads)

continues

continued

- Sodium aluminum sulfate and potassium aluminum sulfate, found in baked goods, packaged goods (such as microwave popcorn), and cheese products
- Sodium benzoate and potassium benzoate, found in sodas
- Bisphenol-A (BPA), found in canned foods. Use fresh, frozen, or dried foods instead.
- Sodium nitrite/nitrate, found in processed meats
- Polycyclic aromatic hydrocarbons (created when fat burns) caused by high heat, such as grilling
- Heterocyclic amines (formed at high temperatures, such as grilling)
- Acrylamide (a carcinogen found in fried foods, chips, crackers, cookies, bread crusts, and toasted cereals)
- Brominated vegetable oil (in fruit-flavored drinks and sodas)
- Dioxins (found in fatty foods). Trim fat from meat (buy grass-fed whenever possible) and avoid non-organic milk.
- Heavy metals (cadmium, lead, aluminum, mercury), found in water, farmed and Atlantic fish, metal and aluminum cans and pans, aluminum foil, paint, teeth fillings, and cigarettes. Drinking lots of fresh, filtered water helps flush the metals from your system.
- Genetically modified organisms (GMOs), found in most processed foods with corn, canola, cottonseed, soy, and sugar beet–based ingredients. Avoid GMOs (which are not labeled) by buying organic foods.
- Polyunsaturated vegetable oils (found in soy, corn, palm oils) are highly sensitive to heat. Use coconut oil naturally refined, expeller-pressed canola oil, butter, or ghee (clarified butter) for high-heat cooking, as they are less susceptible to heat damage. Use extra-virgin olive oil for drizzling on salads and steamed vegetables, and as a bread dip and overall flavor enhancer.
- Soy protein isolate (found in genetically engineered soybeans and not found in organic soy products)
- Artificial sweeteners (aspartame, saccharin, and sucralose)
- High-fructose corn syrup
- Artificial food coloring/dyes (blue 1 and 2, green 3, red 3, and yellow 6)
- MSG (monosodium glutamate), a chemical flavor enhancer

FOODS THAT HURT
AND FOODS THAT HEAL

If you're anything like me, you probably don't appreciate it when some-one tells you to do something but doesn't tell you why you should (or shouldn't) do it. In this "specifics" section, I will explain why certain foods can *cause* pain, whereas others can *fight* pain. Let's start with the "bad" foods and food categories for people with chronic pain.

Seven Foods and Food Categories
That Can Increase Pain

Before you start, I have to tell you that every time I reread this section, I experience a combination of dismay ("I eat so many of these foods") and distress ("I have to change my eating habits"). So, if you are like me, take in the information, start with foods you can eliminate easily ("I can do without soda," for example) and, as with every suggestion in this book, do the best you can. If this all seems overwhelming, on the next page we offer another basic four-week plan to ease you into elimi-nating these harmful foods.

SUGARS: If you eat a lot of sugar and sugar-rich foods, your cells pro-duce a toxic protein-based substance called advanced glycation end products (AGEs). Recognizing the danger, your body works hard to break apart these AGEs by using cytokines, inflammatory messengers that can result in arthritis and other forms of inflammation. Inflamma-tion causes pain, but AGEs can also result in cataracts, heart disease, and wrinkled skin. Try to cut out foods such as candy, sugar-rich des-serts (ice cream, cake, pies, cookies, brownies), sodas (which contain about 10 teaspoons of sugar in every 12-ounce can). Read food labels to search for hidden sugars (corn syrup, fructose, lactose, sucrose, etc.). White bread and white pasta break down quickly into sugar, so try to stay away from those products, too. Our body simply was not designed to break down as much sugar as we consume. Researchers are leaning toward the theory that high blood sugar, which causes an increase in insulin levels, may be the number one cause of heart disease, rather than fat and cholesterol.

Foods That Can Increase Pain

	Week 1	Week 2	Week 3	Week 4
Sugar	Watch out for hidden sugars: corn syrup, fructose, lactose, sucrose, etc.	Eliminate all artificial sweeteners— read labels!	No more sweetened or unsweetened soda!	Avoid low-fat and fruited foods (such as yogurt) that contain extra sugar.
Foods cooked at high temperatures	Gently steam vegetables rather than stir-frying or oven roasting at high temperatures.	Buy a slow cooker and slow cooker recipe book.	Use only glass or microwave-safe ceramic containers in the microwave.	If you use an outdoor grill, use only on low flame to "finish" foods.
Hydrogenated oils	Read labels and learn which foods contain hydrogenated and partially hydrogenated oils.	Buy organic coconut oil for high-temp cooking and stock up on extra-virgin olive oil.	Throw away all packaged microwave popcorn and resolve never to buy movie theater popcorn.	*Always* use butter (grass-fed is best) instead of margarine.
Alcohol	Limit to one drink—now and then.	Read food and medicine labels carefully and avoid products with alcohol added.	In cooking substitute juice or stock for wine.	Substitute cranberry juice with club soda for alcoholic beverages.
Omega-6 fatty acids	Get rid of cooking oils high in omega-6s: corn, cottonseed, grapeseed, safflower, sunflower.	Cut back on chips, crackers, cookies.	Avoid fast foods.	Enjoy nuts as they are high in omega-3s, but in moderation, as they are also high in omega-6s.
Milk and dairy products	Buy a dairy-free cookbook.	Choose sorbet instead of ice cream, gelato, and sherbet.	Substitute Greek yogurt for other kinds of yogurt.	Avoid creamy sauces and soups.
Gluten	Buy a gluten-free cookbook.	Try gluten-free bread, pastas, and cereals.	Check ingredient labels for wheat, barley, and rye.	Buy only deli meats and cheeses labeled gluten-free.

FOODS COOKED AT HIGH TEMPERATURE: Grilled and fried foods also contain AGEs. Save the grill for special occasions and bake or simmer your meats and vegetables. A slow cooker is a great addition to your kitchen—use it as often as possible. (Many of the recipes we offer in the Appendix (see pages 265–292) are cooked in a slow cooker.)

As for microwave ovens, many health coaches and nutritional experts advise avoiding them and using toaster or conventional ovens instead. If you do use a microwave oven, we suggest the following cautions:

- Cover vegetables tightly in a microwave-safe container with a minimal amount of liquid to prevent nutrients from leaching out.
- Do not heat foods in plastic containers or those covered by plastic wrap, as the plastic molecules can leach into your food.
- Use only glass or microwave-safe ceramic containers and cover foods with paper towels or biodegradable waxed paper (dome-shaped microwave covers are another alternative).
- Never stand directly against the microwave while it is heating your food, a caution that is especially important for children whose bodies absorb radiation more easily than adults' do.
- Microwaves often heat food unevenly, so be careful of "hot spots" that might scald your mouth and throat. Again, be especially careful when heating foods for babies and children.
- Take extra care when you boil water in the microwave as it can splatter (eggs cooked in the microwave can also explode on contact with cold air when you open the door).
- Make sure the door and seals on your microwave are not worn or damaged. A faulty microwave may leak radiation. If you're concerned about your microwave, stop using it or contact your state health department, which should be able to test your oven for signs of leakage. (The FDA reports that most microwaves tested do not leak radiation, but at least you will have peace of mind.)

HYDROGENATED OR PARTIALLY HYDROGENATED OILS (TRANS FATS) can damage the cells lining your blood vessels, causing inflammation and intensifying pain. Trans fats are also devastating to your coronary artery system and can increase the risk of heart attacks and strokes. Avoid processed foods whose label or list of ingredients contain the words *partially hydrogenated oils*—margarine, solid vegetable shortening, fried foods (French fries, onion rings, fried chicken, potato chips), fast foods, cookies, frostings, pies, pastries, cakes, doughnuts, crackers, frozen French fries, and packaged microwave popcorn. These products have been subjected to the food-processing equivalent of a nuclear power reactor, getting their atoms bounced around and reconfigured by high heat and complicated chemistry. In this crazy pinball process the atoms realign themselves changing from a natural ("cis") form to an unnatural "trans") form and trans-fatty acids (TFAs) are created. TFAs are believed to be devastating to the coronary arteries and can increase the risk of heart attacks and strokes.

Learn to enjoy healthy fats—avocado, nuts, seeds, coconut oil, extra-virgin olive oil, and pasteurized eggs, grass-fed butter, or ghee from a local dairy or farmers' market.

ALCOHOL: Alcohol is naturally irritating to every cell of your body, especially when you overimbibe. Alcohol-inflamed tissue allows bacteria to pass more easily through the intestinal lining, which leads to irritation and more inflammation. And when alcohol is metabolized, it's basically "instant sugar." Even if you do not have an addiction to alcohol, I strongly recommend eliminating it from your daily diet, or at the very least, limiting your intake to one drink now and then (and by "one drink" I mean a 12-ounce beer, 5-ounce glass of wine, or 1 ounce of hard liquor). But again—better to avoid it completely.

OMEGA-6 FATTY ACIDS, which are plentiful in the average American diet, can increase inflammation and exacerbate pain. It's not that omega-6 fatty acids are bad in and of themselves, but the ratio to omega-3 fatty acids has become seriously unbalanced—human beings evolved with a ratio of 1:1, and the ratio is now 16:1 (with omega-6s on the high end). You can cut down on omega-6 levels by eliminating or cutting back on processed and fast foods and polyunsaturated vegetable oils (soy, corn, sunflower, safflower, cottonseed), which are used in most snack foods, crackers, cookies, and sweets. Seeds and nuts (and the oils extracted from them) also contain omega-6 fatty acids, so if you have arthritis or any type of inflammatory disease, it's best to avoid them. Eat more oily fish (wild salmon, tuna, sea bass, sardines). You can also take fish oil supplements. I have great respect for Dr. Andrew

Weil, who recommends taking a daily fish oil product with 700 to 1,000 mg of EPA (eicosapentaenoic acid) and 200 to 500 mg of DHA (docosahexaenoic acid) in the smallest number of pills.

MILK: Both the sugars and the proteins in milk can trigger arthritis flare-ups, digestive problems, sinus congestion, and headaches. Most people have at least some difficulty digesting milk due to a deficiency of lactase, the enzyme that digests lactose, so cutting milk and dairy products from your diet can actually reduce inflammation and gassiness, indigestion, diarrhea, vomiting, and allergic symptoms, such as a constantly runny nose, skin conditions (eczema, psoriasis), and asthma. Milk is also linked to cataracts, breast cancer, and possibly ovarian cancer. (Restrict your milk intake to limited quantities of local pasture milk, if tolerated.) As for other dairy products, butter and many cheeses have zero carbohydrates and thus zero sugar, and may be well tolerated by some people. Yogurt, which does contain carbohydrates (and therefore sugar), is also often well tolerated because it contains probiotics that help digest lactose. If you can eat dairy yogurt, choose plain Greek yogurt, which is high in protein, but avoid low-fat or fruited yogurts, which tend to be loaded with sugar.

GLUTEN is a protein found in such grains as wheat, rye, barley, and triticale (a cross between wheat and rye). Experts disagree about the percentage of people with gluten sensitivities (an immune reaction to the protein gluten), but a conservative estimate is 6 to 7 percent of the US population—or about 20 million Americans. Some experts believe the figure is as high as 50 percent. People with autoimmune disorders including irritable bowel syndrome, chronic headaches, arthritis, and lupus are at high risk for gluten sensitivity. Symptoms of gluten sensitivity range from digestive problems to headaches, rashes, eczema, fatigue, and mental confusion ("brain fog"). If you think you might have a gluten sensitivity or intolerance, try eliminating all grains and grain products from your diet for a week or two and see whether you feel better. If your symptoms continue, ask your doctor to test you for gluten intolerance or celiac disease, an autoimmune disease that damages the lining of the small intestine, preventing the absorption of some nutrients. Celiac is caused by the body's reaction to eating gluten, which is found in wheat, barley, rye, and possibly oats (which are often cross-contaminated with gluten), and symptoms may include weight loss, bloating, diarrhea, stomach pain, headaches, and fatigue.

Ten Foods That Fight Pain

Now, the good news. The following foods are powerhouses for over-all nutrition and are especially helpful in fighting chronic pain. We include these ingredients in the recipes in the Appendix (see pages 265–292). Try to incorporate these foods into your diet daily. Pick a new food to try every week. Remember, baby steps are okay.

Foods That Fight Pain

	Week 1	Week 2	Week 3	Week 4
Water	Drink at least eight to ten (8-ounce) glasses of water every day.	Buy BPA-free hard plastic water bottles for your car and office.	Research water filtration systems and purchase one that fits your needs and pocketbook.	When you're hungry, always drink a glass of water first, then wait 10 minutes before eating.
Vegetables	Keep a list of the "Clean 15" and "Dirty Dozen Plus" (pages 240–241) and buy organic vegetables whenever possible.	Add a small salad to your lunch or dinner and include veggies on your sandwiches.	Add "greens" to your smoothies—spinach and kale are good choices.	Buy a juicer and experiment with juicing some of the "powerhouse" veggies (add fruit to sweeten the taste).
Fruits	Add cranberries —whole or dried without sugar—to your cereal or in smoothies.	Buy organic apples, red grapes, or cherries and include them with your meals.	Organic blueberries are a real treat—buy (or pick) in bulk in the summer and freeze for the winter.	Try dried or frozen tart cherries in granola, smoothies, or homemade granola bars.

continues

250

Foods That Fight Pain *continued*

	Week 1	Week 2	Week 3	Week 4
Walnuts and almonds	Buy raw, unsalted walnuts and almonds in bulk and store in the refrigerator.	Sprinkle nuts on yogurt, cereal, and salads.	Keep small baggies of these nuts in the fridge for snacks or car trips.	Remember: certified organic, raw, unsalted nuts are best—avoid roasted, sugared, or seasoned nuts.
Seeds	Add chia seeds to yogurt, cereal, or smoothies.	Buy raw, unsalted shelled pumpkin seeds—a healthy snack that contains tryptophan, an essential, sleep-promoting amino acid.	Give flaxseeds a try—they are easiest to digest when ground into meal.	Add raw, shelled hemp seeds to salads, rice, smoothies, cereals, and pancakes.
Extra-virgin olive oil (EVOO)	Buy EVOO in dark, tinted glass bottles.	Store in a cool place, away from light and heat, and use within a year of pressing.	Use EVOO only for low- to medium-heat cooking because of its low "smoke point."	Try organic, cold-pressed hemp seed oil as a substitute for EVOO in salads, pesto, pasta, or bread dips.
Cold-water fish	If you're a fish lover, eat cold-water fish 2–3 times a week.	If you're not a fish lover, try non-fishy fish (cod, halibut, snapper, etc.).	Select wild-caught fish, which tend to be higher in omega-3 fatty acids and protein and are free from antibiotics, pesticides, and artificial dyes as compared to farm-raised fish.	Take an omega-3 fish oil supplement (see suggestions, page 152), especially if you don't eat fish regularly.

continues

Foods That Fight Pain *continued*

	Week 1	Week 2	Week 3	Week 4
Pasture-raised, grass-fed beef and certified organic chicken	Buy these meats whenever possible—even though more expensive, they are much healthier for you.	Grass-fed beef tends to be leaner than grain-fed beef, so be careful not to overcook.	Reduce your meat consumption by eating smaller portions.	Add more fish and vegetarian meals to your weekly diet.
Tea	Try the ginger tea recipe on page 272.	Stock up on oolong, white, or green tea, which are full of health-promoting anti-oxidants.	Try decaffeinated brands, especially if you have trouble sleeping.	Have a cup of soothing, anxiety-reducing, depression-relieving chamomile tea during the day or before bedtime.
Cocoa	Buy raw, certified organic cacao powder and mix with your morning coffee—instant mocha!	Warm up with a cup of hot chocolate: mix 1 cup heated almond milk with 1–2 tablespoons of raw cacao powder and sweeten to taste.	For an extra-special treat, indulge in 70–90% cacao chocolate bars, certified organic, alkali-free.	Try raw, certified organic cacao powder in oatmeal, smoothies, or homemade granola bars (see recipe page 272).

1. WATER: Drinking at least eight to ten 8-ounce glasses of water every day helps the kidneys filter toxins from body fluids and assists the liver in its detoxification duties. Water also helps us to eat less because it "bulks" the food we eat, softening and expanding the food particles, making them easier to digest, and flushing everything through your system quickly and efficiently. Water also makes you feel full so you'll tend to eat less when you drink more. Often when we're hungry, we're actually thirsty! It's a good idea to drink the bulk of your water between meals, as many nutritionists believe that water taken with meals dilutes digestive enzymes, interfering with the digestive process. Sip water during meals and drink lots of water in between meals. If you have a hard time drinking enough water, add slices of lemon, lime, orange, or even cucumber for a refreshing kick.

2. POWERHOUSE VEGGIES include watercress, Chinese cabbage, spinach, parsley, kale, red peppers, broccoli, arugula, cauliflower, and carrots (Google "powerhouse foods" for more choices). These veggies are chock-full of critical nutrients with protective or disease preventive properties and can be eaten raw in salads, or lightly sautéed in olive oil, perhaps with a little garlic. An easy way to get more veggies into your daily meals is to add some to a sandwich or make a small salad to accompany your meal. Smoothies and juices are also easy and delicious ways to get more of these powerhouse foods into your daily diet.

3. FRUITS: *Cranberries*, a powerhouse food, high in dietary fiber, manganese, vitamin K, and vitamin C, are also praised for their anti-inflammatory properties. Tannins in cranberries reduce the ability of bacteria to attach to the urethra and bladder, helping to prevent and treat urinary tract infections. Studies also show that cranberries may help prevent cancer, reduce the risk of heart disease, and promote gastrointestinal and oral health. Buy whole or dried berries processed without sugar and use them in smoothies or trail mix or sprinkled on oatmeal, or drink undiluted (100%) cranberry juice. *Red grapes (organic)* inhibit inflammation and may even help fight cancer. Eating grapes (rather than drinking them) adds fiber and eliminates any added sugar. *Blueberries (organic)* are also an excellent choice, as they are high in phytonutrients with anti-inflammatory and anti-oxidant properties. *Tart cherries* have pain-reducing properties because they contain anti-oxidants, including quercitin, a potent bioflavinoid, and anthocynins, a phytochemical that helps relieve pain more effectively than does aspirin.

4. WALNUTS AND ALMONDS: Walnuts are a terrific source of beneficial omega-3 essential fatty acids and are well known for their anti-inflammatory and cholesterol-lowering effects. Sprinkle them on yogurt, oatmeal, and salads or just grab a handful when you are hungry. Almonds are another good choice as they have more calcium than any other nut and they are rich in fiber and vitamin E, an anti-oxidant that fights inflammation. Avoid roasted, salted, sugared, or seasoned nuts whenever possible. Raw, organic nuts are best.

5. SEEDS: *Chia seeds* are very rich in anti-inflammatory omega-3 fatty acids and, because they slow down your body's conversion of carbohydrates into simple sugars, they can help control blood sugar ups and downs. These tiny seeds are also a potent source of fiber (easier to digest than flax seeds), a powerful digestive aid, and packed full of essential nutrients including proteins, vitamins, and minerals. Sprinkle them on yogurt or cereal, add several tablespoons to your smoothies or protein drink, and use them to thicken soups, gravies, and even meatballs (replacing bread crumbs).

Pumpkin seeds are also chock-full of beneficial nutrients (magnesium, manganese, protein, zinc), phytosterols (beneficial plant compounds), and anti-oxidants. Shelled pumpkins seeds are often labelled "pepitas."

Flaxseeds are high in fiber, omega-3 fatty acids, and phytochemicals called lignans, which reduce the risk of cardiovascular disease and certain cancers. Ground flaxseed (flaxseed meal) is easier to digest than whole.

Hemp seeds are another potent source of omega-3s, as well as a rich source of the essential minerals magnesium, phosphorus, iron, and zinc. Add them to your smoothies, yogurt, or granola.

These four seeds are definitely powerhouse foods, but they pack a caloric wallop if you use them too generously. Per tablespoon, chia seeds have 70 calories, hemp seeds about 60, and flaxseeds about 55. Because these seeds are so fiber rich, when you take them, always be sure to drink lots of water.

6. EXTRA-VIRGIN OLIVE OIL (EVOO) contains a substance called oleocanthol, which interferes with two enzymes (COX-1 and COX-2) that cause inflammation in the body. EVOO also contains polyphenols, which have anti-oxidant and anti-inflammatory properties as well as digestive, bone health, cognitive, and anti-cancer benefits. I strongly suggest you go through your kitchen cabinets and throw out all other oils (except coconut oil and organic, expeller-pressed canola oil, which are safe for high-heat cooking because they are less susceptible than other oils, including EVOO, to heat damage). Be sure to buy "extra-virgin" olive oil ("pure olive oil" is not the same). All oils can go rancid when exposed to light and/or heat, so look for EVOO in dark, tinted bottles (glass, not plastic) and store them in a cool area away from direct (or indirect) heat and light (a pantry is ideal). EVOO is best used within a year of pressing, but it can be safely stored after opening for two to three years. *Do not* use EVOO to heat foods at high temperatures.

7. COLD-WATER FISH: The fatty oils in the fillets and areas around the gut of cold-water fish (wild salmon, albacore tuna, trout, mackerel, herring, anchovies, sardines, smelt, shad) are extraordinarily good for you. Research shows that eating one to two servings of fish every week can reduce inflammation and, thus, pain. Omega-3 fish oil supplements can be used as a substitute if you dislike fish, but many people find that they can acquire a taste for fish by starting out with small helpings of non-fishy fish (cod, grouper, halibut, mahi mahi, snapper, tilapia) and then moving on to cold-water varieties. If at all possible, always select wild-caught versus farm-raised fish.

8. PASTURE-RAISED BEEF AND CERTIFIED ORGANIC CHICKEN: Cows evolved to eat grass and roam the outdoors. "Pasture-raised" refers to where the animal eats—in the pasture and not penned up—and "grass-fed" refers to what it eats. If you're eating beef that's not specifically sold as "pasture-raised" or "grass-fed," you can reliably assume that the cows were penned up for a good part of their lives and fed a high-calorie diet of corn and grain to fatten them up quickly. Corn and grain are full of omega-6 fatty acids, which have been linked to inflammation. Pasture-raised, grass-fed cows are leaner, and their meat is rich in healthy compounds, such as omega-3 fatty acids and vitamin E.

All feed given to USDA-certified organic chickens must be free of pesticides, fertilizers, animal by-products, or other additives and must meet "free range" federal guidelines, with sufficient opportunity to exercise and suitable ventilation and air circulation. Most of the chickens we're offered in supermarkets have spent their lives in close confinement, with food, water, and air piped into their stuffy cages.

Grass-fed beef and free-range chicken are definitely more expensive—but if you ever visit a beef or chicken confinement operation, you will understand why most supermarket meat is less costly. Your best bet is to find local farms and ranches that sell certified organic beef and poultry (as well as eggs and dairy products).

9. TEA: All beverages that are high in water content have anti-inflammatory qualities, and tea is a great choice. White tea, oolong, and green tea are full of catechins, anti-oxidant compounds that reduce artery plaque and inflammation. Tea also has been linked to reduced risk of heart disease, diabetes, and cancer. Be aware that many teas contain caffeine, so if you have trouble with insomnia or if caffeine simply revs you up too much, choose decaffeinated brands. Ginger tea is also a great choice.

10. COCOA: Cocoa contains anti-inflammatory compounds called flavanols, substances that reduce both blood clotting and inflammation in the body. Give yourself a treat and enjoy a weekly cup or two of hot cocoa (make sure it is made with 60 to 70 percent natural cocoa, or cacao). If you're lactose intolerant (and don't like cocoa made with water), try non-dairy milks, such as almond, hemp, oat, rice, and soy milk (be advised that soy is a common allergen). A truly delightful way to enjoy the benefits of natural cocoa is to indulge once or twice a week in an ounce or two of dark chocolate that's at least 70 percent cacao.

A note about omega-3 fatty acids: Many of the "Top 10" foods—flaxseeds, chia seeds, sardines, salmon, beef, and olive oil—are high in omega-3s, conferring an extra bonus. And don't forget eggs! Omega-3-enriched eggs contain three times the omega-3s you'll find in ordinary eggs, because flaxseed or algae are added to the diet of egg-producing hens. Eating three or four enriched, pasteurized eggs every week will help you get your omega-3s even if you are not a fish eater.

SPECIAL DIETARY CONSIDERATIONS

We are all biochemically unique and so there is no such thing as a perfect diet. If you believe you might have food allergies or sensitivities to specific foods or substances (such as salt or specific spices), I strongly suggest you try an elimination diet in which you eliminate a certain food for a period of time—usually two or three weeks—and then slowly reintroduce the food and monitor your symptoms for possible reactions.

Allergy testing can be expensive and results are often unreliable, thus the elimination diet remains the gold standard for identifying specific food allergies or sensitivities.

An anti-inflammatory diet may also help you select and prepare foods that will reduce inflammation, considered a major cause of chronic pain and other chronic diseases, including many cancers, heart disease, and Alzheimer's disease. For the basic principles and details, visit Dr. Andrew Weil's excellent website and search for "anti-inflammatory diet."

Specific Foods for Specific Conditions

I also suggest the following dietary changes for people with specific chronic pain conditions.

If you have arthritis:

- Avoid red meat, poultry, and animal fats, which can inflame your joints.
- Cut back or eliminate "nightshade" veggies (eggplants, peppers, tomatoes, potatoes).
- Avoid oranges and orange juice (the acids in oranges can irritate delicate joint membranes).
- Gamma linoleic acid (GLA), an essential fatty acid found in borage oil, evening primrose oil, and black currant oil, has anti-inflammatory properties. As always, ask your doctor or health-care professional for advice when taking dietary or herbal supplements.

If you have chronic fatigue syndrome or fibromyalgia (which many experts believe have a common cause and may represent the same underlying disorder):

- You may have food allergies, so schedule an appointment with a physician or nutritionist for assessment.
- Avoid red meat and dairy products and eat only organic fish and chicken; choose "wild" fish over farm-raised fish, if possible.
- Limit or eliminate sugar, honey, corn syrup, and sugar substitutes.
- Avoid fried, greasy, and highly processed foods, and avoid caffeine, which paradoxically drains energy from your depleted system.

If you have chronic head and neck pain:

- Be sure to drink lots of water, especially if you feel a headache coming on.
- Flax- and chia seeds are high in omega-3s and can fight the inflammation that causes headaches; krill oil (krill are shrimplike crustaceans) is one of the most potent sources of omega-3s, but because of possible drug interactions, use only under a physician's supervision.
- Ginger has anti-inflammatory properties and can ease migraine-related nausea.
- Small doses of caffeine can sometimes help with headaches, but too much caffeine can trigger them.

If you have diabetes:

- Stop eating sugar and refined carbohydrates and avoid overeating.
- Eliminate red meat from your diet and always remove skin from poultry.
- Drastically reduce or eliminate dairy products.
- Increase your intake of fatty fish (wild salmon, sardines, herring, mackerel, bluefish, albacore tuna).

On pages 265–292, you'll find some of our favorite recipes for every meal. These recipes incorporate many of the tips and principles discussed throughout this chapter. We've included these to help ease you into the kitchen and back to health—in the most delicious way possible!

All you need is love.
But a little chocolate now and then doesn't hurt.

—CHARLES M. SCHULZ

ELEVEN

FINAL WORDS

Awareness, Courage, Diligence, Hope, Faith, Joy, Compassion, and Wonder

Find a place inside where there's joy,
and the joy will burn out the pain.

—JOSEPH CAMPBELL

The key to living—and thriving—with chronic pain lies not outside you but within you, in the power you can generate within your own body, mind, and spirit to reinvigorate your energy and enthusiasm for life. Your strength arises from an acceptance of some measure of pain as part of your life and, from there, your willingness to learn about and tap into your innate healing potential.

In this final chapter we outline the essential "ingredients" in the Pain Antidote formula. For the proper alchemy to work, we believe that all these components are necessary. With a commitment to foster and nurture your internal resources, we are convinced that you will succeed.

AWARENESS

When you know better, you do better.

—MAYA ANGELOU

You can't change something—a behavior, thought, or emotion—if you don't know it is happening. Seeing the truth of what's going on inside and outside of you is the key to changing it. Being gentle and nonjudgmental as you learn about yourself is essential for you to be successful. Awareness of the present moment, one breath at a time, is a crucial part of the antidote.

COURAGE

Freedom lies in being bold.

—ROBERT FROST

A key component of pain recovery is change—and change can be scary. A litany of "what ifs" might stand in your way. Letting go of the familiar with no assurance that you will be okay is one of the big problems you will face every day. Walking through your fear takes courage, but the brave energy you bring to this process will change your life for the better.

DILIGENCE

What we hope to do with ease,
we must learn first to do with diligence.

—SAMUEL JOHNSON

To be successful, you will need to work hard. This book is filled with suggestions to guide you on your journey, but learning to be persistent, attentive, and conscientious does not come easily or naturally to any of us. Take a good look at the Jump Start Plan in Chapter 9 and choose the techniques you are willing to engage in with commitment and purpose—then get to work and be diligent!

HOPE

I feel so much better since I gave up hope.

—ZEN COMIC BOOK

Hope can promise more than it can deliver. Hope can move you from reality into illusion. So, I believe in "measured hope." Perhaps as a teaspoon of sugar sweetens the bitter taste of coffee, so can a bit of hope lighten up your day. Still, you wouldn't want to put a teaspoon of coffee into a cup of sugar and swallow it. Life, reality, whatever we call what "is" right now, in the moment, is not always easy and may, in fact, be downright awful. Sweetening the "awful" with a sprinkling of hope won't hurt you. But be careful not to live in that sugar bowl. Drowning in sweetness and light may be worse than treading water in the dark.

FAITH

None of us knows what might happen
even the next minute, yet still we go forward.
Because we trust. Because we have Faith.

—PAULO COELHO

I recall an old story about a man who is hanging from a ledge with a tiger growling down and preventing him from climbing up. Although a non-believer, he decides to throw caution to the wind and looking up at the heavens, he calls out: "If there's anyone up there, please help me! I'll do anything if you save me!!" He hears a booming voice from above that says, "Let go!"

He stares at the tiger, then contemplates the chasm below before shouting, "Is there anyone else up there?"

Faith is assuming there is some force greater than you that will help. Whether that force is a religiously conceived image or a simple amorphous belief really doesn't matter. As Anne Lamott writes, "Faith is noticing the mess, the emptiness and discomfort, and letting it be there until some light returns."

JOY

You've gotta dance like there's nobody watching,
Love like you'll never be hurt,
Sing like there's nobody listening,
And live like it's heaven on earth.

—WILLIAM W. PURKEY

Living with chronic pain managed by powerful drugs destroys joy. Awakening to the beauty around you, living fully in the present moment, is a catalyst for joy. You need only to breathe deeply to find the moment and appreciate it—all of it. I've recently started to pay close attention to the joy of taking a hot shower at the end (in addition to the beginning) of the day and counting my blessings as I let the soothing, healing water rain down on me.

Discover the places where you find joy in simple pleasures.

COMPASSION

Love and compassion are necessities, not luxuries.
Without them, humanity cannot survive.

—DALAI LAMA XIV

So many people with chronic pain are isolated and extremely hard on themselves. We feel as if we have somehow failed and are undeserving of love and support from others. The healing process consists of easing off the "beating yourself up" attitude that has become part of our daily lives. When we are kind toward ourselves, our approach to life and to others becomes lighter and more connected. The antidote to aloneness is compassion, first toward ourselves, and then toward others. It is this soft, gentle approach that we have attempted to offer you throughout this book and which we encourage you to continue to nurture as you proceed through your recovery. Loving compassion, or loving-kindness, is a sustaining force that will lead you from darkness to the light.

WONDER

Wonder is the experience of mystery. It is a fascinated
recognition of great beauty where a moment before we
noticed only routine; it is an attitude of amazement
and perplexity, and sometimes a stunned curiosity in the
face of the astonishing and inexplicable. In some way,
however strange, it is often a form of homage elicited
by the presence of something larger than ourselves.

—PAUL BROCKELMAN

We can do no better than to end this book with a story that personifies
a sense of wonder at the beauty and mystery of life—and, at the same
time, encompasses all the other components of the antidote: awareness,
courage, diligence, hope, faith, joy, and compassion, as well as love.

Gary D'Agostino, 58, is dying.

An automotive service manager for years and a steam engineer by
trade, "Dag" became addicted to OxyContin, fentanyl, and other opioid drugs after numerous rugby injuries, race car crashes, and a near-
fatal motorcycle accident that shattered fifteen bones in his body. Pain
was his constant companion.

Knowing that Dag was addicted to the drugs prescribed for him for
his chronic pain and fearing that the massive doses might kill him, his
wife, Liz, organized an intervention. Three hours later ("the sun had
barely shifted its position," Dag laughs, remembering), he was on a
plane headed to treatment at LVRC.

"For the next ten days I used all my intellectual powers to go through
the motions to satisfy the staff, knowing that when I got home I'd start
all over again," Dag recalls. "But then something happened. The earth
shifted, I had that moment of clarity that everyone who loved me had
hoped and prayed for. I knew I was exactly where I needed to be, exactly when I needed to be there. And that's when I literally rolled up
my sleeves and committed myself to the program, filling myself with
the opportunities presented to me. Whatever they were willing to give
to me, I was willing to accept. It was a profound experience. I became
an honor student, a best pupil."

After completing the twenty-eight-day program, Dag returned home clean, sober, and firmly committed to recovery. But for some reason that his doctors couldn't figure out, he kept losing weight. Even when he was put on a daily 4,000-calorie diet, he lost weight. Something was gravely wrong, but no one could diagnose him.

Four months and dozens of tests later, Dag's doctor solemnly announced the diagnosis: Dag had amyotrophic lateral sclerosis (ALS), often referred to as "Lou Gehrig's disease," a progressive, degenerative neurological disease that affects nerve cells in the brain and the spinal cord. The median survival time from onset to death is thirty-nine months.

Dag figures he has at least a few years left in him. "I have a terminal disease, and I don't know when I'll check out," he says matter-of-factly. "But here's the deal—I'm going to do my level best every day. I refuse to allow this disease to identify me. Compared to addiction, ALS is a walk in the park. I don't know how long I have to live, but going through the process of recovery has given me the strength and the tools that I need to deal with the challenges of ALS. That's the crazy thing about this—there is absolutely no way I could have handled ALS if I hadn't gone through treatment for chronic pain and addiction."

Dag is a philosophical person who loves to talk about the mysteries and miracles of life. "It's so real and so absolute and so tangible," he says, his words tripping over themselves, "that if treatment can work for me, as screwed up as I am, and turn me around to be able to face this stuff with grace and courage, then it can work for anybody. However the recovery process functions in other people's lives, if you can find the key to unlocking that door to clarity, the rest will fill in. It's all about finding that key. For me, the key was understanding for the first time the depth and breadth of the love, trust, and faith of my family and friends. I would not allow that to be wasted. I couldn't. I just could not allow that to be wasted. And when I found that key, that's when the fear went away forever, that's when the shame and the guilt went away. All of that was lifted. That was the moment of surrender."

Sitting in his wheelchair on the patio in his backyard, Dag says, "I'm sick and I'm going to die. That's okay, I can deal with that. But I'll be damned if I'm going to check out of this life in the throes of addiction.

"The last two years when I have been able to walk in recovery have been the best years of my life. I have been able to live—to live! If the disease takes me tomorrow, I can turn around and say, 'You know what? I did the best I could. And I am happy.'"

Dag is quiet for a moment, staring at the trees in his yard, a slow smile spreading across his face. "Did you know that there are twenty-three shades of green in my backyard? I counted them. That's something I never would have done when I was taking drugs and in constant pain. I wouldn't even have seen those trees; they would just be a blur. But I spent a whole afternoon out here, just looking at the different shades of green.

"And I counted them all," he said, smiling broadly. "Imagine that."

Delicious and Nutritious
Pain-Reducing Recipes

Here are some of our favorite meal suggestions. Many of these recipes were given to us by LVRC patients, who also suggest three small electrical appliances that will make your life in the kitchen much easier: a 4- to 6-quart slow cooker, an immersion blender, and an egg cooker.

We've included many slow cooker recipes to make your life in the kitchen less stressful—these recipes are marked with a slow cooker symbol ▮ . Lightly greasing the slow cooker with olive oil cooking spray or coconut oil will make cleanup a lot easier.

An immersion blender will allow you to blend soups right in the slow cooker rather than your needing to transfer the hot soup in batches to a standing blender.

Egg cookers offer a foolproof way to hard-boil eggs (up to ten at a time)—great for a quick snack or sliced on salads. Most models include a tray for poaching eggs, and some include an additional tray to make omelets for a quick and easy meal. Be sure to buy organic, pasture-raised eggs whenever possible.

A few important notes:

- Whenever possible, buy organic. Refer back to the list on page 241 of the "Dirty Dozen Plus" fruits and vegetables that are loaded with pesticides and should always be bought "100% organic."
- Extra-virgin olive oil is our favorite oil, but for cooking at medium-high heat (searing meat or fish, stir-frying), use coconut oil; organic, expeller-pressed canola oil; or organic ghee (clarified butter), all of which have a medium-high smoke point. Ghee is available in many health or whole food stores.
- Use olive oil cooking spray to lightly grease the slow cooker—it will make cleanup much easier!
- Seeds and nuts are most healthful when purchased raw, organic, and unsalted.

- Use filtered or purified water whenever possible. A reverse osmosis filter on your sink is a great addition to your kitchen.
- If you are in recovery from alcohol addiction and do not want to use vanilla or almond extracts (which contain slight amounts of alcohol), use imitation vanilla, which is alcohol-free. You can also replace the extract with an equal amount of pure maple syrup.
- Several recipes ask for parchment paper, which is located next to the aluminum foil and waxed paper in your grocery store.

RECIPES

Beverages and Breakfast

Salads and Sides

Desserts

Beverages and Breakfast

Banana-Blueberry-Cranberry Smoothie

SERVES 2

Double the recipe and store extra in the fridge for lunch or a snack.

1 banana, peeled and cut in half (frozen works!)
¼ cup frozen organic blueberries
¼ cup dried or fresh cranberries
2 tablespoons chia seeds
2 cups chilled unsweetened vanilla-flavored almond milk

Blend all the ingredients in a blender for 30 seconds, or until combined.

Creamy Coconut Oatmeal

SERVES 10 TO 12

Cook overnight and breakfast will be ready for you in the morning. Serve with chia seeds, pumpkin seeds, and dried or fresh organic fruit, such as cranberries, blueberries, or strawberries.

Olive oil cooking spray
2 cups organic steel-cut oats
1 (13.5-ounce) can organic coconut milk
1 teaspoon vanilla or almond extract
Honey, raw organic agave nectar, or pure maple syrup

1. Grease a slow cooker with olive oil cooking spray. Place 8 cups of water and the oats, coconut milk, and vanilla in the slow cooker. Cook on LOW overnight or for about 8 hours, until creamy.
2. Sweeten with honey, agave, or maple syrup if desired.
3. Store leftovers in the fridge for up to a week.

Homemade Almond Creamer

MAKES 1 CUP CREAMER

Make your own coffee creamer—no additives or preservatives! You'll need a blender and a nut milk bag (available in kitchen stores or online) or clean kitchen towel. Stored in refrigerator, this will keep for three or four days. You can also use the leftover almond pulp in dozens of recipes—just search online for "almond pulp recipes."

1 cup raw almonds, organic if possible
1 to 2 cups water (purified or filtered is best), plus more for soaking
Dash of vanilla or almond extract
Honey, maple syrup, or raw organic agave syrup (optional)

1. Soak the almonds overnight or longer (up to 48 hours) in cold water in an airtight container. If soaking longer than overnight, change the cold soaking water every 12 hours or so.
2. After soaking drain the almonds and rinse again with purified water.
3. Place the soaked almonds and 1 to 2 cups of fresh purified water in a blender. Blend for about a minute.

4. Place the nut milk bag over a bowl or large measuring cup, carefully empty the almond mixture into the bag, and gently squeeze the bag with your hands.
5. Flavor with the vanilla. If desired, sweeten the almond creamer with honey, maple sugar, or agave.
6. Store in the fridge (mason jars are great for storage). The cream will separate slightly—no worries, just shake before using. Use within 3 to 4 days for best taste.

Variation:
Try flavoring with ½ teaspoon of raw cacao powder for a mocha flavor.

Lots-of-Energy Crackers

MAKES 30 CRACKERS

These nutty, ultra-nutritious crackers are great for a snack—or spread with almond butter, peanut butter, or hummus for a quick breakfast or lunch.

½ cup chia seeds
½ cup raw, unsalted sunflower seeds
½ cup raw, unsalted pepitas (pumpkin seeds)
½ cup sesame seeds
1 large garlic clove, finely grated
1 teaspoon grated sweet onion
Optional: Season with kosher or sea salt, rosemary,
    and/or freshly ground black pepper

1. Preheat the oven to 325°F. Line a large baking sheet with parchment paper.
2. Mix the seeds together in a large bowl.
3. In a small bowl, combine 1 cup of water with the garlic and onion and whisk together for a minute or so. If desired, add ½ teaspoon of salt, 1 teaspoon of rosemary, and/or ½ teaspoon of black pepper to the water mixture.
4. Pour the water mixture onto the seeds and stir until thick and combined.
5. Spread the mixture on the prepared baking sheet with the back of a spoon until it's less than ¼ inch thick. If it's too thin, just patch it up with your fingers.
6. Bake for 30 minutes. Remove from the oven, score into 1½- to 2-inch squares, and carefully flip onto the other side, using a spatula. Bake for 25 minutes or perhaps a bit more—watch carefully to make sure the

crackers are a light golden color on the bottom. Bake longer if you like crispy crackers.

7. Allow to cool completely on the pan. Store in the fridge in a sealed container or resealable plastic bag.

No-Fail Popovers

MAKES 8 TO 10 POPOVERS

If you are not gluten- or dairy-free, these popovers are a real treat, super easy to make, and very impressive with their puffed-up tops.

Butter or coconut oil, for pan
1 cup sifted all-purpose flour
¼ teaspoon kosher or sea salt
2 large organic, pasture-raised eggs
1 cup cold milk

1. Grease eight to ten wells of a popover or muffin tin and set aside.
2. Beat the eggs in a medium-size bowl, then sift flour and salt over the eggs. Add the milk and beat the mixture until smooth.
3. Fill the wells of the prepared muffin tins two-thirds full.
4. Place in a *cold* oven; set the oven to 450°F.
5. Bake for 30 minutes, until browned on top.

Oatmeal Pancake à la Markus

SERVES 1

This is Dr. Pohl's favorite weekend breakfast. Top with no-sugar applesauce, pure maple syrup, or fruit.

1 cup organic steel-cut oats
6 large organic, pasture-raised egg whites (see note)
¼ teaspoon vanilla extract
1 to 2 tablespoons chia seeds
1 teaspoon ground cinnamon
1 tablespoon olive oil or olive oil cooking spray

1. Place all the ingredients, except the oil, in a medium-size bowl. Whisk for 1 to 2 minutes until smooth.

2. Heat the oil in a medium-size pan over medium-low heat.
3. Pour the mixture into the pan, cover, and cook until lightly browned, 3 to 4 minutes.
4. Flip over to brown the other side, about 2 minutes.

Note: Check out YouTube videos for quick and easy ways to separate egg whites from yolks.

Sausage, Hash Browns, and Egg Casserole

SERVES 12

A great company dish and perfect for holidays and large family gatherings. Cook overnight for an easy, delicious breakfast feast in the morning!

Olive oil cooking spray
1 pound nitrate-free sausage
1 onion, chopped
1 organic bell pepper (green, red, or orange), seeded and chopped
1 tablespoon extra-virgin olive oil
1 (32-ounce) bag frozen, gluten-free hash brown potatoes
1½ cups shredded Cheddar cheese
12 large organic, pasture-raised eggs
1 cup whole milk
½ teaspoon kosher or sea salt
½ teaspoon freshly ground black pepper

1. Spray the inside of a slow cooker with olive oil cooking spray.
2. In a small skillet, brown the sausage, then drain well. (Tip: rinsing the sausage with hot water before draining removes a lot of the fat.)
3. Clean the pan and heat the olive oil. Cook the onion and bell pepper until crisp-tender. Let cool for 5 to 10 minutes.
4. Place one third of the frozen hash brown potatoes in the prepared slow cooker. Add one third each of the sausage, onion and pepper mixture, and cheese. Repeat the layers, ending with the cheese.
5. In a large bowl, beat the eggs, milk, and seasonings until well mixed. Pour over the ingredients in the slow cooker and cover.
6. Cook on LOW for 10 to 12 hours, until the casserole is set and the eggs are thoroughly cooked. (If you have a new, hotter-cooking slow cooker, this may take only 8 to 9 hours; the eggs should reach a temperature of 160°–165°F.)

Variations:
- If you are vegetarian, substitute veggie crumbles for the sausage.
- Havarti or Swiss cheese can be substituted for the Cheddar.
- Add some minced chiles or jalapeño peppers if you like spicy food.

Slow Cooker Ginger Tea

MAKES 2 QUARTS

This tea keeps well in the refrigerator for two to three weeks (store in a sealed container), and it is just as good hot or cold—either way gives you the healing and anti-inflammatory benefits of this power root. Be sure to add fresh lemon or lime slices later, when you are ready to drink.

2 to 3 cinnamon sticks
8 to 10 thin slices peeled fresh ginger (more won't hurt!)
Lemons or limes, sliced
Honey or raw organic agave nectar, to sweeten (optional)

1. Place 2 quarts of water and the cinnamon and ginger in a slow cooker. Cook on LOW for 2 to 3 hours.
2. Ladle into cups and add lemon slices.
3. Sweeten with honey, if desired.

Variations:
- If the ginger taste is a bit strong for you, mix the tea with warm water.
- For mint ginger tea, add fresh mint to the tea for 5 minutes at the end.

Slow Cooker Granola Bars

MAKES 10 LARGE- OR 15 MEDIUM-SIZE BARS

Great for breakfast, snacks, lunch on-the-go—or even dessert!

1½ cups organic steel-cut oats
¼ cup flax meal
¼ cup unsweetened shredded coconut
2 tablespoons chia seeds
½ teaspoon baking powder
½ teaspoon kosher or sea salt
½ cup pure maple syrup

2 teaspoons vanilla or almond extract
⅓ to ½ cup coconut or almond butter, softened
2 large, organic, pasture-raised eggs
4 to 5 chopped organic dates, figs, or prunes
Olive oil cooking spray

1. Combine the oats, flax meal, coconut, chia seeds, baking powder, and salt in a large bowl. Mix well.
2. Combine the maple syrup, vanilla, coconut butter, and eggs in another bowl. Mix well.
3. Add the wet ingredients to the dry and mix until combined. Fold in the dates.
4. Grease a slow cooker with olive oil cooking spray. Place parchment paper in the bottom and up the sides of the greased slow cooker, to create a sling with which to remove the baked mixture.
5. Spoon the batter into the prepared slow cooker and pat the mixture down well so it's evenly distributed.
6. Cook on LOW for about 2½ hours, or until the middle of the mixture is solid (not mushy); let cool in the slow cooker for 20 to 30 minutes.
7. Use the edges of the parchment paper to lift and remove the mixture. Set aside to cool for 30 to 40 minutes.
8. Cut the mixture into bars, using a pizza cutter.
9. Store the bars in the refrigerator or freeze them.

Slow Cooker Omelet

SERVES 4–6

Great for brunch, as the omelet takes only a few hours to cook.

10 large organic, pasture-raised eggs
½ teaspoon dry mustard
½ teaspoon salt
½ teaspoon freshly ground black pepper
1½ cups diced ham, Canadian bacon, or veggie crumbles
Olive oil cooking spray
1½ cups Cheddar cheese
½ cup chopped green onions or green bell pepper
Chopped fresh parsley, for garnish

1. Whisk the eggs in a large bowl.
2. Add the mustard, salt, and pepper. Stir in the ham.

3. Oil a slow cooker with olive oil cooking spray. Pour the egg mixture into the prepared slow cooker.
4. Sprinkle the cheese and green onions over the top of the egg mixture.
5. Cover and cook on HIGH for 1½ to 2 hours or on LOW for 2½ to 3 hours, or until the eggs are set but not overcooked.
6. Garnish with the parsley sprigs.

Variation: Add one of the following herbs (all which go well with eggs) to the egg mixture before cooking: basil, chives, dill, or thyme, or paprika.

Vegetarian Soups and Meals

Asparagus and Spinach Risotto

SERVES 4

Risotto cooked on the stove is time-consuming. This vegetable-rich risotto makes for a filling lunch or light dinner and can be assembled in minutes and on the table in just a few hours.

2 tablespoons extra-virgin olive oil
4 shallots, diced
1½ cups arborio rice
1 to 2 garlic cloves, crushed
4 cups vegetable or chicken stock
Kosher or sea salt and freshly ground black pepper
10 to 15 asparagus spears, cut into ½-inch lengths
8 ounces organic baby spinach leaves
½ cup regular or vegan Parmesan cheese

1. Heat the oil in a skillet, add the shallots, and sauté over medium heat, stirring, for 2 to 3 minutes.
2. Add the rice and garlic and cook for 2 additional minutes, stirring. Add ½ cup of the stock and let boil for 30 seconds.
3. Transfer the rice mixture to a slow cooker, add the remaining 3½ cups of stock, and season to taste with salt and pepper. Cover and cook on HIGH until the liquid is absorbed, about 2 hours.

4. Stir the cut-up asparagus into the rice mixture, then spread the spinach over the top. Cover and cook on HIGH for an additional 30 minutes, until the asparagus is just tender and the spinach is wilted.
5. Sprinkle with the Parmesan cheese and serve.

Billy's Black Bean Stew

SERVES 4 TO 6

As Billy says, "I just eat it and eat it and eat it and can't wait to make it again." Top with your choice of chopped tomatoes, red onion, parsley, cilantro, grated cheese, and/or avocado., and serve with crusty bread and a simple organic spinach salad topped with pomegranate seeds and your favorite dressing.

2 tablespoons olive oil
8 ounces smoked tofu, cut into small cubes (about 1 cup cubes)
1 small onion, finely chopped
2 large carrots, peeled and finely chopped
1 red (or green) bell pepper, finely chopped
1 sweet potato, cut into small cubes
2 garlic cloves, minced
2 teaspoons ground cumin
1 teaspoon paprika
1 teaspoon dried oregano
1 (15-ounce) can black beans, drained and rinsed
3 cups low-sodium vegetable broth (more if you want a soup rather than a stew)
Kosher or sea salt and freshly ground black pepper

1. Heat 1 tablespoon of the olive oil over medium heat in a medium-size saucepan, add the tofu cubes, and cook until the tofu is browned and crispy, 8 to 10 minutes. Remove the tofu from the pan and set aside.
2. In the same pan, heat the remaining 1 tablespoon of olive oil. Add the onion, carrots, bell pepper, and sweet potato. Sauté over medium heat until the vegetables are soft, 5 to 10 minutes. Add the garlic and stir for 30 seconds, then add the cumin, paprika, and oregano and cook, stirring, for another 30 seconds.
3. Add the black beans, broth, and salt. Bring the stew to a boil, lower the heat to low, and simmer uncovered for 30 minutes, or until most of the liquid has evaporated. Mash some of the black beans, using the back of a wooden spoon. Add the reserved tofu and cook for another 5 minutes.

Curried Butternut Squash Soup

SERVES 4

A terrific lunch soup or as a starter for a dinner party—the recipe can easily be doubled (but be sure to use a larger soup pot).

  1 large butternut squash
  1 tablespoon extra-virgin olive oil
  1 onion, diced
  2 teaspoons curry powder
  2 cups low-sodium vegetable or chicken broth
  1 (13.5-ounce) can light coconut milk
  Kosher or sea salt and freshly ground black pepper

1. Preheat the oven to 350°F. Cut the squash in half, scooping out and discarding the seeds, then cut into quarters and place on a baking sheet. Roast in the oven for 25–30 minutes, or until soft. Remove from the oven and let cool.
2. Sauté the onion in the olive oil in a 2-quart saucepan over medium heat. When translucent, add the curry powder and stir for about 5 minutes, cooking the curry until it is fragrant.
3. Add the squash in spoonfuls to the onion mixture.
4. Add the broth and bring to a simmer. Cook until squash is so soft it falls apart, about 10 minutes. Remove from the heat and let cool.
5. Add the coconut milk and puree the mixture in the saucepan with an immersion blender. Warm through.
6. Add salt and pepper to taste.

Variation: Add ½ to 1 additional teaspoon of curry powder for a stronger curry flavor.

Hearty Split Pea Soup

SERVES 6 TO 8

This delicious soup is chock-full of veggies. Serve with sourdough or gluten-free bread.

  Olive oil cooking spray
  4 cups dried split peas, rinsed
  6 cups organic, low-sodium vegetable or chicken broth

2 cups diced white or sweet potatoes
2 celery stalks, chopped
2 to 3 large carrots, chopped
1 medium-size onion, chopped
½ teaspoon dried thyme or marjoram
2 bay leaves
½ teaspoon basil
2 to 3 garlic cloves, finely chopped
1 teaspoon kosher or sea salt
Freshly ground black pepper

1. Spray a slow cooker with olive oil cooking spray. Combine all the ingredients in the prepared slow cooker, cover, and cook on LOW for 8 to 12 hours.
2. Uncover and turn the heat to high, then simmer until the soup reaches your desired consistency.

Variations:
- Stir in ½ teaspoon of red pepper flakes or 1 teaspoon of curry powder.
- Use half broth and half water.
- If you are not vegetarian, try adding 1 cup of diced ham or 4 slices of Canadian bacon, cut into small pieces.

Rustic Roasted Tomato Soup

SERVES 4

If you grow tomatoes in the summer, chances are you'll be looking for recipes to handle the abundance! This rich, flavorful soup will become a summer favorite—and it doubles as a pasta sauce! For a simple side dish, slice an avocado and top with walnuts or unsalted sunflower seeds with a splash of balsamic vinaigrette dressing.

4 cups chopped tomato
2 garlic cloves, smashed
½ teaspoon fennel seeds or 1 teaspoon Italian seasoning
5 tablespoons olive oil
Kosher or sea salt and freshly ground black pepper
4 sprigs fresh basil
1½ to 2 cups country-style bread, such as baguette or ciabatta, crust removed, that has been torn into 2-inch pieces

1. Preheat the oven to 450°F.
2. Toss the tomato, garlic, fennel seeds, and 3 tablespoons of the oil in a large baking dish; season with salt and pepper.
3. Roast the tomato mixture in the oven about 45 minutes, stirring occasionally, until the tomatoes are browned and the juice thickens.
4. Transfer the tomato mixture to a large saucepan. Add the basil, 1 cup of the bread, and 4 cups of water.
5. Bring to a boil, lower the heat, and simmer until the bread is softened and the soup has thickened, 8 to 10 minutes. Season with salt and pepper.
6. While the soup simmers, cut the remaining bread into smaller pieces, toss on a baking sheet with the remaining 2 tablespoons of oil, season with salt, and toast in the oven, tossing often, until crisp, 5 to 8 minutes.
7. Serve the soup topped with the toasted bread.

Sweet Potato Lentil Soup

SERVES 4

This hearty soup can easily serve as a main meal with bread and a simple organic greens salad topped with pomegranate seeds or dried cranberries.

2 tablespoons coconut oil
1 medium-size or 2 small onions, diced
1 teaspoon finely minced fresh ginger, or ¼ teaspoon ground
1 teaspoon ground turmeric
1 teaspoon ground cumin
½ teaspoon cinnamon
⅛ teaspoon cayenne pepper
¼ teaspoon kosher or sea salt
2 to 3 medium-size sweet potatoes, peeled and cut into ¾-inch cubes (2 to 3 cups)
4 cups low-sodium vegetable broth
2 (14.5-ounce) cans diced tomatoes, with the juice
1 cup dried pink or red lentils (rinse and pick over carefully)

1. Heat the oil in a large pot over medium heat. Sauté the onion in the oil for 2 to 3 minutes, until soft and slightly translucent. Stir in the ginger and cook for 2 to 3 additional minutes. Add the turmeric, cumin, cinnamon, cayenne, and salt.
2. Add the sweet potatoes, broth, tomatoes and their juice, and lentils.
3. Bring to a boil, lower the heat, cover, and simmer for 30 minutes or so.

Meat- and Fish-Based Meals

Baked Shrimp Scampi

SERVES 6

This recipe is a bit complicated but it's worth the effort, especially for company or a special family dinner. Serve with quinoa and steamed broccoli.

2 pounds (24–30 medium-size) shrimp, peeled and deveined
3 tablespoons coconut oil
Kosher or sea salt and freshly ground black pepper
12 tablespoons (1½ sticks) unsalted butter, at room temperature
4 to 6 teaspoons minced garlic (4 to 6 cloves)
¼ cup minced shallots or finely diced onion
¼ cup minced fresh parsley leaves
1 to 2 teaspoons minced fresh rosemary leaves
¼ teaspoon crushed red pepper flakes
1 teaspoon grated lemon zest
2 tablespoons freshly squeezed lemon juice
1 extra-large organic, pasture-raised egg yolk
⅔ cup panko bread crumbs
Lemon wedges, for serving

1. Preheat the oven to 425°F.
2. Place the shrimp in a medium-size bowl and toss gently with the coconut oil, 1 teaspoon of salt, and ½ teaspoon of pepper. Allow to sit at room temperature while you make the butter and garlic mixture.
3. In a small bowl, mash the butter with the garlic, shallots, parsley, rosemary, red pepper flakes, lemon zest, lemon juice, egg yolk, bread crumbs, ½ teaspoon of salt, and ¼ teaspoon of pepper until combined.
4. Remove the shrimp from the coconut oil mixture and arrange them in a large, oval baking dish.
5. Pour the remaining coconut oil marinade over the shrimp.
6. Spread the butter mixture evenly over the shrimp, using your hands to arrange evenly.
7. Bake for 10 to 12 minutes, until hot and bubbly. If you would like the top to be browned, place under a broiler for 1 minute.
8. Serve with lemon wedges.

Buttery Turkey Breast

SERVES 8 TO 10

Who said turkey is just for the holidays?

1 (6- to 7-pound) bone-in turkey breast
Kosher or sea salt
¼ teaspoon freshly ground black pepper
½ teaspoon dried rosemary
½ teaspoon dried thyme
8 tablespoons (1 stick) butter, cut into 2-tablespoon chunks

1. Wash the turkey breast and pat dry. Season lightly with the salt, pepper, rosemary, and thyme.
2. Place in a slow cooker, dot with the butter, and cook on LOW for 10 to 12 hours.

Variation: For a less-butter option, rub the turkey with just 2 tablespoons of softened butter. Put 1 cup of chicken broth in the slow cooker, then add butter-rubbed turkey.

Chicken Piccata

SERVES 6 TO 8

A very impressive company dish! Serve with organic red grapes and steamed broccoli or asparagus.

Olive oil cooking spray
4 large boneless chicken breasts
1½ cups brown rice flour
2 tablespoons extra-virgin olive oil
¼ to ½ cup freshly squeezed lemon juice
6 tablespoons nonpareil capers (see note)
1½ cups chicken broth
½ teaspoon freshly ground black pepper

1. Spray a slow cooker (see note) with olive oil cooking spray.
2. Cut the chicken breasts in half lengthwise (don't worry if the halves aren't equal).

3. Put the flour in a bowl and dredge both sides of the chicken in the flour.
4. Heat the olive oil in a skillet (nonstick is okay, cast iron or heavy-bottomed is better) over medium heat.
5. Brown the chicken on both sides, about 2 minutes per side. (You'll need to do this in batches.)
6. Place the chicken, lemon juice, capers, broth, and pepper in the prepared slow cooker.
7. Cook on LOW for 4 to 6 hours or on HIGH for 2 to 3 hours, until the chicken is cooked through and the sauce has thickened.

Notes:

You'll need a 4- to 6-quart cooker for this dish—if your slow cooker is smaller, halve the recipe.

Nonpareil capers are smaller and more delicate in taste and flavor. *Nonpareil* means "has no equal" in French.

Cook-Ahead Chicken for Quick Meals

MAKES 4 TO 5 CUPS CHICKEN

This cook-ahead chicken recipe makes life much easier when a recipe calls for chicken in soup, salads, pasta dishes, or casseroles.

Olive oil cooking spray
4 large boneless chicken breasts (see note)
½ cup gluten-free chicken stock or water

1. Spray a 4-quart slow cooker with olive oil cooking spray. Put the chicken breasts in the prepared slow cooker (see note).
2. Pour the stock over the chicken.
3. Cook on HIGH for 3 to 4 hours or on LOW for 6 to 7 hours.
4. Put the chicken and its broth in the refrigerator for up to 3 days, or freeze breasts in a resealable plastic bag or sealed container for up to a month.

Note: Keep the breasts whole (don't cut into pieces) to help retain moisture.

Garlic and Lime Fish Fillets Baked in Foil

SERVES 4

Lime juice, cinnamon, and garlic spice up this delicious fish dish. Serve with green salad with walnuts, feta, and pears (page 288).

4 serving-size pieces fish (cod, rockfish, halibut, or salmon)
½ teaspoon kosher or sea salt
Freshly ground black pepper
¼ cup extra-virgin olive oil
¼ cup raw organic agave nectar
Lime juice from 2 large or 3 small limes
Pinch of ground cinnamon
1 red onion, sliced
4 scallions, sliced
6 garlic cloves, chopped

1. Preheat the oven to 350°F.
2. Tear off eight pieces of foil, two for each piece of fish.
3. Place one serving of fish on a piece of foil; season each serving with salt and pepper.
4. Combine the olive oil, agave, lime juice, and cinnamon in a measuring cup and pour the mixture over the fish pieces. Be careful to fold up the edges of the foil to catch any overflow.
5. Sprinkle the fish with the onion, scallions, and garlic.
6. Place the remaining pieces of foil on each serving and fold the edges together to create a packet.
7. Bake for about 20 minutes, or until the fish flakes easily but isn't dried out.

Roast Chicken with Artichokes

SERVES 4

A zesty roast chicken—this recipe definitely requires a 6-quart slow cooker! Serve kale or organic greens sprinkled with feta cheese and walnuts or seeds (pumpkin or sunflower seeds). Use the carcass to make homemade chicken stock for soup the next day (recipe follows).

Olive oil cooking spray
1 medium-large onion, quartered
1 large carrot, sliced

1 (3- to 4-pound) chicken
1 large lemon, halved
4 or more garlic cloves, peeled
1 to 2 tablespoons extra-virgin olive oil
½ teaspoon dried rosemary
½ teaspoon kosher or sea salt
½ teaspoon freshly ground pepper
1 (6-ounce) jar marinated artichoke hearts

1. Grease a 6-quart slow cooker with olive oil cooking spray.
2. Place the quartered onion and carrot slices in the prepared slow cooker.
3. Remove any innards from the chicken. Rinse off the chicken; pat dry with a paper towel.
4. Put one-half of the lemon and all the garlic cloves into the cavity of the chicken.
5. Place the chicken on top of the veggies in the slow cooker.
6. Cut the rest of the lemon into large slices and place the lemon slices on top of the chicken.
7. Drizzle the olive oil over the bird, and sprinkle with rosemary, salt, and pepper.
8. Cook on LOW for 6 to 8 hours or on HIGH for 3 to 4 hours.
9. About an hour before serving, drain the artichokes and place them on top of the chicken and continue cooking in the slow cooker.

Variation: For chicken stew, add 2 large celery stalks, sliced, and 3 to 4 white, red, or sweet potatoes. After cooking remove roast chicken from pot, remove meat from carcass, and stir meat into the pot. Eliminate the artichoke hearts.

Homemade Chicken Stock

MAKES 6 TO 8 CUPS STOCK

So easy to make, so much healthier than store-bought stock, and so great to have on hand when a recipe calls for chicken broth or stock.

Chicken carcass and any leftover juices and veggies from previous recipe
1 onion, roughly chopped
1 celery stalk with leaves, roughly chopped
1 carrot, roughly chopped (no need to peel)
2 bay leaves
Fresh parsley, thyme, rosemary, and/or sage
1 to 2 teaspoons kosher or sea salt

1. After you remove the meat from the freshly cooked chicken, put the bones back in the slow cooker, along with the cooking juices.
2. Add the onion, celery, carrot, bay leaves, herbs, and salt on top of the bones and fill the slow cooker with water, leaving a margin of ½ to 1 inch at the top.
3. Cook on LOW for 8 to 10 hours or overnight.
4. Strain the entire contents of the pot through a colander (you may need help with this as slow cookers can be heavy) with a large soup pot underneath.
5. Discard the solids and chill the stock in the refrigerator overnight, until a fat layer accumulates on the top. Remove the fat.
6. The stock can be refrigerated for 3 to 4 days—or freeze for up to 3 months in mason jars or other sealed containers, being sure to leave 1 inch at the top for expansion.

Salmon with Creamy Avocado-Mint Sauce

SERVES 4

Mix cool mint with hot jalapeño and you've got a great combination of flavors, perfect for summer suppers. Serve with corn on the cob and fresh tomato and cucumber slices.

    1 avocado, peeled and pitted
    1 cup lightly packed fresh mint leaves
    ½ cup 2% Greek yogurt
    ½ jalapeño pepper, seeded
    Juice of ½ lemon
    1 teaspoon kosher or sea salt
    ½ teaspoon freshly ground black pepper
    1 to 2 tablespoons organic ghee or organic, expeller-pressed canola oil
    4 (4- to 6-ounce) salmon fillets

1. Puree the avocado, mint, yogurt, jalapeño, lemon juice, salt, and pepper in a food processor.
2. Heat the ghee or oil in a large skillet over medium-high heat.
3. Season the salmon with salt and pepper. Sear, flesh side down, until just cooked through, about 6 minutes. Lower the heat if the fish is sticking to the pan. Discard the skin (a sharp knife gently scraped against the flesh makes quick work of this).
4. Top the salmon with the sauce.

Slow Cooker Beef Stew

SERVES 4 TO 6

The V8 juice is a surprise ingredient in this healthy, vegetable-packed slow cooker stew. Serve with sourdough bread for a warm and filling meal.

- 1 to 2 pounds stew beef
- ½ cup all-purpose flour
- 2 to 3 tablespoons extra-virgin olive oil
- 4 to 5 red potatoes, peeled and cut into quarters
- 2 to 3 carrots, cut into chunks
- 1 to 2 celery stalks
- 1 onion, chopped into medium-large pieces
- 1 pound mushrooms, sliced or quartered
- ½ to 1 teaspoon kosher or sea salt
- ½ teaspoon freshly ground black pepper
- 1 to 2 bay leaves
- 1 (16-ounce) can low-sodium V8 vegetable juice
- ½ cup water or beef broth

1. Dredge the beef in the flour (use a sealed plastic container and be sure to shake off any extra flour before browning).
2. Heat the oil in large skillet over medium heat, add the beef chunks, and brown lightly on all sides.
3. Place all the ingredients in a slow cooker in this order: potatoes, carrots, celery, beef, onion, mushrooms, salt, pepper, bay leaf, V8 juice, and water.
4. Cover and cook on HIGH for 4 hours or on LOW for 8 to 9 hours. If the stew looks soupy, leave the lid off for 15 to 20 minutes before serving.

Turkey and Brown Rice Chili

SERVES 4 TO 6

A super-easy recipe when you don't have much time before dinner. Serve with bread and a simple arugula salad with your favorite dressing.

- 1 pound ground turkey
- ¼ cup chopped onion
- Olive oil cooking spray
- 1 (14-ounce) can diced tomatoes

1 to 2 tablespoons chili powder
1 to 2 teaspoons chopped garlic
1 teaspoon ground cumin
1½ cups water or organic, low-sodium chicken broth
1 cup cooked brown rice
1 (15-ounce) can organic kidney beans, drained and rinsed

1. Brown the turkey in a large skillet, 5 to 6 minutes, or until cooked through. Add the onion and cook until softened, 2 to 3 minutes.
2. Spray a slow cooker with olive oil cooking spray. Spoon the browned turkey mixture into the oiled slow cooker; add all the remaining ingredients, except the cooked rice and the beans. Cover and cook on HIGH for 2 to 3 hours or on LOW for 5 to 6 hours.
3. Stir in the rice and beans about an hour before serving; cover and continue to cook in the slow cooker until heated through.

Variation: Add extra chili powder or red pepper flakes if you like really "hot" chili.

Salads and Sides

Broiled Tomatoes with Parmesan

SERVES 2

Even if you are not a tomato fan, this recipe will win you over. We use organic, expeller-pressed canola oil instead of extra-virgin olive oil because of the high cooking temperature.

4 beefsteak or other large, juicy tomatoes
2 tablespoons organic, expeller-pressed canola oil
¼ cup freshly grated Parmesan cheese, or to taste
2 tablespoons chopped fresh parsley

1. Preheat the broiler.
2. Core the tomatoes, cut in half, and place in pie pan or shallow roasting pan.
3. Using a tablespoon or small measuring cup, drizzle each tomato with canola oil.
4. Spoon the cheese on top—a little or a lot!

5. Broil 5 inches from the heat, watching carefully, until the tomatoes are golden brown, 3 to 4 minutes.
6. Sprinkle with the chopped parsley.

Buttery Carrots and Red Potatoes

SERVES 6 TO 8

What could be prettier than orange carrots and red potatoes as a side dish? You may want to double the carrots—they shrink as they cook and they're so delicious, they disappear fast when served. This is Kathy's go-to company side dish, and she's never had leftover carrots.

8 tablespoons (1 stick) butter, sliced into 1-tablespoon pats
8 organic red potatoes, cut in half
1 (1-pound) bag organic baby carrots
Fresh parsley

1. Preheat the oven to 375°F.
2. Divide the butter slices equally between two roasting pans; heat in the oven until melted, being careful not to burn the butter.
3. Remove the pans from the oven; place potatoes, cut side down, in one pan and cook for 20 minutes; then place the carrots in the other pan and put both pans back in the oven.
4. Brush every 15 minutes or so with butter from the pan—you may want to add more butter—and cook for an additional 30 to 40 minutes, until the potato "faces" are browned and crispy and the carrots are soft.
5. Sprinkle with the parsley.

Cauliflower "Mashed Potatoes"

SERVES 4

These aren't real mashed potatoes, of course, but they taste great and have a fraction of the calories and all the health benefits of a powerhouse vegetable.

1 medium-size head cauliflower
1 bay leaf
1 tablespoon minced garlic
½ teaspoon kosher or sea salt
¼ teaspoon freshly ground black pepper

1 tablespoon cream cheese, softened
¼ cup grated Parmesan cheese
½ teaspoon chopped fresh chives, or dried, for garnish
Unsalted organic butter

1. Clean the cauliflower, cutting off the stems, then cut into quarters and place in a slow cooker. Fill the slow cooker with water until it covers the cauliflower.
2. Add the bay leaf, garlic, salt, and pepper to the pot.
3. Cover and cook on HIGH for 4 hours or on LOW for 6 hours—test to make sure the cauliflower is very tender.
4. Remove the lid, drain off all the water, and discard the bay leaf.
5. Add the cream cheese and Parmesan to the pot and mash, using a potato or rice masher.
6. Garnish with the chives. Serve with butter, if desired.

Variations:
- For the cream cheese, substitute 1 tablespoon of olive oil.
- Substitute fresh rosemary or chopped scallions for the chives.

Green Salad with Walnuts, Feta, and Pears

SERVES 4 TO 5

This is Kathy's favorite salad for special dinners or potlucks. Simple to make and yet filled with complex flavors. The amounts listed are approximate—adjust to your taste (more pears, less feta, etc.).

2 medium-size, ripe organic pears, peeled or unpeeled
3 tablespoons freshly squeezed lemon juice
1 head butter, red, or green leaf lettuce, cleaned and dried
1½ to 2 tablespoons extra-virgin olive oil
½ cup coarsely chopped walnuts
½ to 1 cup feta cheese
1 to 2 teaspoons red wine vinegar
Freshly ground black pepper

1. Cut the pears into thin slices, place in a small bowl, and cover with the lemon juice.
2. Tear (gently!) the lettuce into bite-size pieces, place in a medium-large salad bowl, and pat dry with paper towels once again. Drizzle lightly with the oil and toss.

3. Mix in the walnuts and feta, sprinkle with the vinegar, and add pepper to taste. Toss gently.
4. Using a slotted spoon or fork, lift the pear slices out of the bowl of lemon juice and arrange on top of the salad.

Lemon-Garlic Green Beans

SERVES 4

A colorful side dish, perfect with Buttery Turkey Breast (page 280) or Chicken Piccata (page 280).

Olive oil cooking spray
1½ pounds fresh green beans, ends trimmed
3 tablespoons extra-virgin olive oil
3 large shallots, diced
6 garlic cloves, minced
1 tablespoon grated lemon zest
½ teaspoon kosher or sea salt
½ teaspoon freshly ground black pepper
½ cup water or chicken broth
Sliced almonds, for garnish

1. Spray a 4-quart slow cooker with olive oil cooking spray. Put the green beans in the prepared slow cooker and top with the remaining ingredients, except the almonds.
2. Cook on LOW for 6 to 8 hours or on HIGH for 3½ to 4 hours. The beans will be crispy—if you like softer beans, cook for an extra hour. (Extra cooking time doesn't equal mushy beans—they're sturdy vegetables and can withstand cooking for a long time.)
3. Serve with sliced almonds.

Sweet, Sweet Potato Fries

SERVES 4 TO 6

Just a tablespoon (or two) of sugar caramelizes the potato wedges—you might need to double the recipe, these are so good!

3 large sweet potatoes
3 to 4 tablespoons organic, expeller-pressed canola oil or organic ghee

1 tablespoon kosher or sea salt
1 to 2 tablespoons organic brown sugar
1 to 2 tablespoons paprika or Chinese five-spice powder (or try a mixture of both)

1. Preheat the oven to 450°F. If you want super-crispy fries, you can bump up the heat to 500°F. Put a baking pan in the oven so it is nice and hot when the potatoes are ready to cook.
2. Peel the sweet potatoes and cut off the pointy ends. Cut into rounds, or if you prefer wedges, cut in half crosswise, then in half lengthwise, then crosswise again to make thick wedges. Sweet potatoes are very dense and hard to cut, so use a sharp knife and watch your fingers!
3. Put the potato pieces in a large bowl, add the oil and mix well to combine. Sprinkle with the salt, sugar, and spices. Use your hands to mix well so all pieces are well coated.
4. Spread the potato pieces in a single layer on the hot baking sheet (you may need to bake in batches). No need to oil the pan (but you can always use olive oil cooking spray if you want to avoid a messy cleanup).
5. Bake for 15 minutes, remove the pan from the oven, turn over all the pieces, and return the pan to the oven. Bake for another 10 to 15 minutes, or until the fries are nice and brown, even crispy. They'll be hot, so let cool for 5 minutes before serving.

Zucchini with Butter and Parmesan

SERVES 4

So easy and so good—the Parmesan melts into the zukes to create a veggie dish even children love.

3 to 4 small zucchini, thinly sliced
2 tablespoons butter
¼ cup Parmesan or Romano cheese

1. Steam the zucchini until soft.
2. Toss with the butter and Parmesan.

Desserts

Sugar isn't our best friend, but if you limit your sugar intake to an occasional after-dinner treat—and avoid sugar-rich sodas and snacks during the day— there's no real harm done. Just be mindful and indulge sparingly!

Cranberry-Peach-Apple Crumble

SERVES 4

Mixing tart cranberries with sweeter fruits (apples, peaches, pears) adds up to a scrumptious dessert—and with no eggs or dairy, this recipe is a vegan delight.

Coconut oil or vegan shortening, for pan
2 cups total organic apples and pears, cored and sliced or cubed
½ cup whole organic cranberries, frozen and slightly thawed
1 to 2 tablespoons raw, organic agave syrup
1½ teaspoons ground cinnamon
1 teaspoon arrowroot starch
1 cup gluten-free flour or pancake mix (see variation)
¾ cup organic light brown sugar
Pinch of ground nutmeg
1 to 2 tablespoons coconut oil or water

1. Preheat the oven to 350°F.
2. Grease a deep 9-inch pie plate or 8-inch square baking dish with coconut oil.
3. Toss the apple and pear pieces with the slightly thawed cranberries in a medium-size bowl. (If you use fresh cranberries, they may be a bit crunchy—but still yummy!)
4. Drizzle the fruit with the agave, sprinkle with ½ teaspoon of the cinnamon and the arrowroot, and stir to coat.
5. In a separate bowl, combine the flour, brown sugar, remaining teaspoon of cinnamon, and the nutmeg and coconut oil. Use your hands to mix the ingredients into a soft, coarse crumble.
6. Sprinkle a few tablespoons of the crumble mixture into the bottom of the prepared pan. Spoon in the fruit mixture and top with the remaining crumble mixture, spreading evenly.
7. Bake at 350°F in the center of the oven for 35 to 45 minutes, or until the filling is bubbly and the top is golden brown.

8. Let cool for 15 to 20 minutes. Serve warm (can also be served at room temperature).
9. Cover and refrigerate the leftovers.

Variation: Use ½ cup of gluten-free flour mix and ½ cup organic steel-cut oats.

Gluten-Free Peanut Butter Cookies

MAKES 14 TO 18 COOKIES

These soft and yummy cookies are gluten- and dairy-free.

1 cup organic no-stir peanut butter
1 cup organic light or dark brown sugar
2 teaspoons vanilla or almond extract
⅔ cup oat flour
1 teaspoon baking soda
⅛ teaspoon kosher or sea salt
¼ cup water or almond milk

1. Preheat the oven to 350°F. Line a baking sheet with parchment paper.
2. In a large bowl, cream together the peanut butter and brown sugar for 1 minute. Add the vanilla and mix for another 30 seconds.
3. In a separate bowl, mix together the oat flour, baking soda, and salt.
4. Slowly add the dry ingredients to the peanut butter mixture, mixing well until the dough is crumbly.
5. Add the water or milk and mix until just incorporated—don't overmix.
6. Roll the dough into balls (1½ to 2 tablespoons per cookie), drop 2 inches apart on the parchment-lined baking sheets, and flatten with a fork one way and then the other to create a crisscross pattern.
7. Bake for 8 to 10 minutes, or until just starting to turn golden on the edges (they bake fast, so watch them carefully).

Variation: If you like chewy cookies, add another ⅓ cup of oat flour.

Resources

Our Resources section is simple and straightforward. Rather than fill these pages with so many suggestions that you wouldn't know where to begin, we have carefully selected the books, CDs/DVDs, and online resources that we believe are most helpful for those searching to expand their understanding of chronic pain, opioids, addiction, and recovery. We divide these resources into parts 1, 2, and 3 to align with the topics covered in the corresponding sections of the book and list them alphabetically by title.

PART 1: UNDERSTANDING

Recommended Reading

A Day Without Pain by Mel Pohl (Central Recovery Press, 2011)

Anatomy of an Illness: As Perceived by the Patient, 20th anniversary edition, by Norman Cousins (W. W. Norton, 2005)

Back in Control by David Hanscom (Vertus Press, 2012)

Back Sense: A Revolutionary Approach to Halting the Cycle of Chronic Back Pain by Ronald Siegel, Michael Urdang, and Douglas Johnson (Harmony, 2002)

Being Sober: A Step-by-Step Guide to Getting To, Getting Through, and Living in Recovery by Harry Haroutunian (Rodale, 2013)

Beyond the Influence: Understanding and Defeating Alcoholism by Katherine Ketcham and William F. Asbury (Bantam, 2000)

Brain Rules by John Medina (Pear Press, 2008)

Buddha's Brain by Rick Hanson with Richard Mendius (New Harbinger, 2009)

The Emotional Life of Your Brain by Richard Davidson and Sharon Begley (Plume, 2013)

The Gift of Pain by Paul Brand and Philip Yancey (Zondervan, 1997)

Learned Optimism: How to Change Your Mind and Your Life, by Martin Seligman (Vintage, 2006)

On Death and Dying by Elisabeth Kübler-Ross (Scribner, 2014)

Pain Recovery: How to Find Balance and Reduce Suffering From Chronic Pain by Mel Pohl, Frank Szabo, Daniel Shiode, and Robert Hunter (Central Recovery Press, 2009)

Pain Recovery for Families: How to Find Balance When Someone Else's Chronic Pain Becomes Your Problem Too by Mel Pohl, Frank Szabo, Daniel Shiode, and Robert Hunter (Central Recovery Press, 2010)

The Recovery Book: Answers to All Your Questions About Addiction and Alcoholism and Finding Health and Happiness in Sobriety, revised edition, by Al Mooney, Catherine Dold, and Howard Eisenberg (Workman, 2014)

Some Assembly Required: A Balanced Approach to Recovery from Addiction and Chronic Pain by Dan Mager (Central Recovery Press, 2013)

There Is a Solution: The Twelve Steps and Twelve Traditions of Pills Anonymous (Pills Anonymous World Service Office, 2013)

Under the Influence: A Guide to the Myths and Realities of Alcoholism by James Milam and Katherine Ketcham (Bantam, 1983)

Websites

www.brainrules.net
www.instituteforaddictionstudy.com
www.thepainantidote.com
www.williamwhitepapers.com

DVDs

Pleasure Unwoven: A Personal Journey About Addiction by Kevin McCauley (Institute for Addiction Studies)

PART 2: OVERCOMING

Recommended Reading

Acceptance and Commitment Therapy for Chronic Pain by Joanne Kelly Wilson, Carmen Luciano, and Steven Hayes (Context Press, 2005)

A Gradual Awakening by Stephen Levine (Anchor, 1989)

Changing Course: Healing from Loss, Abandonment, and Fear by Claudia Black (Hazelden, 2002). NOTE: If you are a family member of someone struggling with addiction or chronic pain, we highly recommend all of Claudia Black's books.

Chi Kung in Recovery: Finding Your Way to a Balanced and Centered Recovery by Gregory Pergament (Central Recovery Press, 2013)

Experiencing Spirituality: Finding Meaning Through Storytelling by Ernest Kurtz and Katherine Ketcham (Tarcher/Penguin, 2014)

Feeling Good: The New Mood Therapy by David Burns (Harper, 2008)

The Feeling Good Handbook by David Burns (Plume, 1999)

The Five Elements of Self-Healing: Using Chinese Medicine for Maximum Immunity, Wellness, and Health by Jason Elias and Katherine Ketcham (Harmony, 1998)

Forgive for Good: A Proven Prescription for Health and Happiness by Fred Luskin (HarperCollins, 2002)

Help Thanks Wow: The Three Essential Prayers by Anne Lamott (Riverhead 2012). Anything written by Anne Lamott is high on our list.

Mindfulness-Oriented Recovery Enhancement for Addiction, Stress, and Pain by Eric Garland (NASW Press, 2013)

No More Letting Go: The Spirituality of Taking Action Against Alcoholism and Drug Addiction by Debra Jay (Bantam Dell, 2006)

No More Sleepless Nights by Peter Hauri and Shirley Linde (Wiley, 1996)

Not God: A History of Alcoholics Anonymous by Ernest Kurtz (Hazelden, 1979)

The Recovering Body: Physical and Spiritual Fitness for Living Clean and Sober by Jennifer Matesa (Hazelden, 2014)

The Road Less Traveled: A New Psychology of Love, Traditional Values and Spiritual Growth by M. Scott Peck (Touchstone, 2003)

The Spirituality of Imperfection: Storytelling and the Search for Meaning by Ernest Kurtz and Katherine Ketcham (Bantam, 1992)

Start Where You Are: A Guide to Compassionate Living by Pema Chödrön (Shambhala, 2001). This is our favorite Pema Chödrön book, but we highly recommend all her books and audio CDs.

Yoga for Emotional Balance: Simple Practices to Help Relieve Anxiety and Depression by Bo Forbes (Shambhala, 2011)

Yoga for Pain Relief: Simple Practices to Calm Your Mind and Heal Your Chronic Pain by Kelly McGonigal (New Harbinger, 2009)

Websites

www.greatergood.berkeley.edu The Greater Good Science Center at University of California, Berkeley, "studies the psychology, sociology, and neuroscience of well-being, and teaches skills that foster a thriving, resilient, and compassionate society." The website offers free online courses, a video series, recommended books, and much more.

www.marc.ucla.edu The Mindful Awareness Research Center at UCLA offers free guided meditations, including a 12-minute body scan meditation for sleep.

For Help Quitting Smoking

American Cancer Society offers an excellent "Guide to Quitting Smoking" on its website: www.cancer.org
Toll-free hotline: 1-800-ACS-2345 (1-800-227-2345)

American Heart Association offers numerous resources on its website: www.
heart.org/heartorg/
Toll-free number: 1-800-242-8721

American Lung Association offers a comprehensive, interactive "Quitter In
You" website: www.quitterinyou.org
Toll-free hotline: 1-800-LUNGUSA (1-800-586-4872)

CDs

3 Meditations to Live By (Rod Stryker)

Guided Meditations for Difficult Times: A Lamp in the Darkness (Jack Kornfield).
This CD includes a "forgiveness" meditation.

Guided Mindfulness Meditation (Series 1, 2, 3) (Jon Kabat-Zinn)

Healthy Sleep (Andrew Weil and Rubin Naiman)

Meditations for Emotional Healing: Finding Freedom in the Face of Difficulty (Tara
Brach)

Mindfulness Meditation for Pain Relief (Jon Kabat-Zinn; includes body scan)

Relaxation Body Scan and Guided Imagery for Well-Being (Carolyn McManus)

*The Pema Chödrön Audio Collection: Pure Meditation, Good Medicine, From
Fear to Fearlessness* (Pema Chödrön)

PART 3: MOVING FORWARD

Recommended Reading

*Eating for Recovery: The Essential Nutrition Plan to Reverse the Physical Damage
of Alcoholism* by Molly Siple (Da Capo, 2008)

Eating Right to Live Sober by Katherine Ketcham and L. Ann Mueller (Ma-
drona, 1983)

Foods That Fight Pain: Revolutionary New Strategies for Maximum Pain Relief by
Neal Barnard (Three Rivers, 1998)

*Full Catastrophe Living: Using the Wisdom of Your Body and Mind to Face
Stresses, Pain, and Illness* by Jon Kabat-Zinn (Bantam, 2013)

How Can I Help: Stories and Reflections on Service by Ram Dass and Paul Gor-
man (Knopf, 1985)

It Takes a Family: A Cooperative Approach to Lasting Sobriety by Debra Jay (Hazelden, 2014)

Peace is Every Step: The Path of Mindfulness in Everyday Life by Thich Nhat
Hanh (Bantam, 1992)

Acknowledgments

We owe an enormous debt of gratitude to our extraordinarily talented editor, Renée Sedliar. Renée is an author's dream editor—insightful, intuitive, responsive, gifted with a sense of humor and a profound love of the written word, and deeply involved at every point in the writing of the book. We cannot adequately express our gratitude for the time and energy she so enthusiastically devoted to this book. We are also indebted to Iris Bass, copyeditor; Claire Ivett, editorial assistant; Sean Maher, marketing director; Amber Morris, project director; and the entire Da Capo Perseus team.

Heartfelt thanks to our delightful and resourceful literary agent Linda Loewenthal, who recognized the promise of this book and worked hard to help us craft a strong proposal. Linda's gifts extend far beyond the difficult work of "agenting"—she is a supremely gifted editor who is devoted to excellence in every project she represents. We also owe Linda many thanks for her expert guidance in helping us select Da Capo Press as our publisher.

For offering words of wisdom to share with readers on healing methods and strategies, we thank: George Arias, physical therapist; Rich Bakir, chiropractor; Lynda Christenson, masseuse; Jason Elias, acupuncturist and herbalist; Robin Hamilton, yoga instructor; Elaina Jensen, psychiatric-mental health and certified addiction nurse practitioner; Greg Pergament, Chi Kung instructor; Cheryl Slader, yoga and Reiki instructor; and Marika Tomkins, health coach.

We are grateful to Eduardo Vazquez for his superb acupoint illustrations and his willingness to work under intense deadline pressure.

For their encouragement, support, generosity of spirit—and most of all for graciously sharing their lives with us—we are deeply indebted to Amy Ayoub, Jane and Ed Barragar, Claudia Black, Will Brown, Lenna Buissink, Mikey Chambers, Diana Churchill-Bailey, Joe Cruse and Sharon Wegscheider-Cruse, Robert and Carol Cutrer, Gary and Liz D'Agostino, Dan and Lori Edney, Tilak Fernando, Laura Fitzsimmons, Chooch Gavin, Debbie Goodeve, Paul Groce, Sheila Hagar, Kristen and James Hamilton, Gary Hamman, Billy Heath, Jackie, Isaac and Orion Hindawi, Delbert and Kathleen Hutchison, Debra and Jeff Jay, Julie Johnson, Denny Kay, Irene Kay, Kevin Kelly, Jody Davies Ketcham, Michael Ketcham, Ernest Kurtz, John Lambrose, Maggie Lambrose, John Lanzillotta, Allison Lyons, Jennifer Matesa, D Meyerson, Marla Morrell, Lisa, Naomi and Oron Nadiv, Arthur Newkirk, George Perkins, Amy Pitt, Larry and Vida Pohl, Judy Ranan, Rita Ranan, Kekau Rosehill, Gary Schroeder, Greg Shay, Cheryl Slader, Donn Smith, Alison Spencer, Benjamin Spencer, Patrick Spencer, Robyn Spencer, Joyce Sundin, Alice and Patti Sykes, Jodie Trafton, Sharon Wegscheider-Cruse, William L. White, and Mike York.

We are grateful to the teachers from whom we learned so much: Pema Chödrön, His Holiness the Dalai Lama, David Hanscom, Jon Kabat-Zinn, Jack Kornfield, Ernest Kurtz, Stephen and Ondrea Levine, Barry Rosen, Thich Naht Hanh, Jodie Trafton, and the inspiring group of like-minded docs.

A special thank you to each and every one of the dedicated professionals at the Las Vegas Recovery Center, including but not limited to Stuart Smith, Johanna O'Flaherty, Kristine and George Gatski, Dan Shiode, Debbie Champine, and all of the counselors, nurses, clinical associates, and support staff.

Finally, we dedicate this book to the best teachers of all: OUR COURAGEOUS PATIENTS AND FRIENDS

Index